KU-242-598

OXFORD MEDICAL PUBLICATIONS

MPS selected chapters from
the Oxford Handbook of
Clinical Examination
and Practical Skills

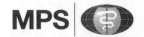
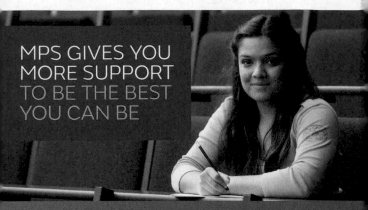

MPS selected chapters from the Oxford Handbook of

Clinical Examination and Practical Skills

2nd edition

Edited by

Dr James Thomas
Consultant Musculoskeletal Radiologist
Nottingham University Hospitals NHS
Trust, Nottingham, UK

and

Dr Tanya Monaghan
Academic Clinical Lecturer in Gastroenterology
NIHR Nottingham Digestive Diseases Centre Biomedical
Research Unit,
Nottingham University Hospitals NHS Trust,
Nottingham, UK

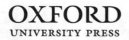
OXFORD
UNIVERSITY PRESS

OXFORD
UNIVERSITY PRESS

Great Clarendon Street, Oxford, OX2 6DP,
United Kingdom

Oxford University Press is a department of the University of Oxford.
It furthers the University's objective of excellence in research, scholarship,
and education by publishing worldwide. Oxford is a registered trade mark of
Oxford University Press in the UK and in certain other countries

© Oxford University Press 2014

The moral rights of the authors have been asserted

First Edition published in 2007
Second Edition published in 2014

Impression: 2

This edition (containing chapters 1, 2, 3, 18, 19 & 20 from the *Oxford Handbook of
Clinical Examination and Practical Skills 2nd Edition*) first printed 2014

Published in the United States of America by Oxford University Press
198 Madison Avenue, New York, NY 10016, United States of America

British Library Cataloguing in Publication Data
Data available

Library of Congress Control Number
Data available

ISBN 978–0–19–872819–1

Printed in Italy by
L.E.G.O. S.p.A.—Lavis TN

Oxford University Press makes no representation, express or implied, that the drug
dosages in this book are correct. Readers must therefore always check the product
information and clinical procedures with the most up-to-date published product
information and data sheets provided by the manufacturers and the most recent
codes of conduct and safety regulations. The authors and the publishers do not
accept responsibility or legal liability for any errors in the text or for the misuse or
misapplication of material in this work. Except where otherwise stated, drug dosages
and recommendations are for the non-pregnant adult who is not
breast-feeding.

Links to third party websites are provided by Oxford in good faith and
for information only. Oxford disclaims any responsibility for the materials
contained in any third party website referenced in this work.

Preface to the main edition

Since the publication of the first edition of this book, we have been heartened by the many positive comments and emails from readers and have been very grateful for the suggestions for improvements and modifications. We have tried to incorporate as many of these as possible.

We have tried hard to update the text to reflect modern practice and to make changes which, only with the 20–20 vision of hindsight, could we see were needed.

We have tried to keep an eye on OSCE examinations and the reader will find new 'skills stations' throughout the book to add to the existing examination frameworks.

Several chapters, including respiratory, paediatrics, skin, and locomotor have been rewritten from scratch.

We have incorporated new chapters on the eyes, the obstetric assessment.

The 'important presentations' section of each systems chapter has been greatly expanded and referenced to our sister publications the *Oxford Handbooks Clinical Tutor Study Cards*.

The practical procedures chapter has been significantly expanded and updated.

The photographs throughout the book have been updated to reflect modern healthcare dress codes.

There is a brand new chapter on 'other investigations' so that the reader can understand what is involved in common tests and how to prepare patients for them.

Finally, the chapter order has been changed to highlight the importance of the 'core' system examinations of the cardiovascular, respiratory, abdominal, and nervous systems.

As always, we welcome any comments and suggestions for improvement from our reader—this book, after all, is for you.

James D Thomas
Tanya M Monaghan
2013

Acknowledgements to the main edition

We would like to record our thanks to the very many people who have given their advice and support since the publication of the first edition.

For contributing specialist portions of the book, we thank Dr Caroline Bodey (Paediatrics), Dr Stuart Cohen (Skin, hair, and nails), Dr John Blakey (Respiratory), Dr A Abhishek (Locomotor) and Mr Venki Sundaram and Mr Farid Afshar (Eyes).

Once again, the elderly pages have been penned by the peerless Dr Richard Fuller who remains a steadfast supporter and is much appreciated.

This edition builds on the work of contributors to the first edition whose efforts deserve to be recorded again. Thanks then to Heid Ridsdale, Franco Guarasci, Jeremy Robson, Lyn Dean, Jonathan Bodansky, Mandy Garforth, and Mike Gaell.

For this edition, Michelle Jie, Muhammad Umer, and Dr Sandeep Tiwari kindly posed for new and updated photographs. Their bravery made the process easy and enjoyable. Our continued gratitude goes to our original models, Adam Swallow, Geoffrey McConnell, and our anonymous female model. We thank the staff at the Nottingham University Hospitals Medical Photography Department, in particular Nina Chambers for taking the photographs.

Additional diagrams for this edition, including the skin pictures, have been drawn by Dr Ravi Kothari and we thank him for his speedy and high-quality work.

As well as contributing some material for the procedures chapter, Dr Yutaro Higashi has remained a grounding force during this process. His wisdom and sagely advice throughout have been much appreciated.

Finally, we would like to thank the staff at Oxford University Press for originally trusting us with this project, especially Catherine Barnes and Elizabeth Reeve for their faith, support, and guidance.

Contents

How MPS can help you through your studies

Medical Protection (MPS) – More than defence for students

Congratulations from all of us at MPS on becoming a student of medicine!

We hope you find your first Oxford handbook a useful tool, one of many as part of your membership benefits.

You may be wondering, who we are, what we do and why you've joined us.

Medical Protection is the world's leading defence organisation for doctors. More than 70% of medical students in the UK are members, and we protect and support more than 300,000 members in the UK and beyond.

Whilst it's unlikely that, as a medical student, you'll need our medicolegal assistance, most medical schools will ask you to be a member of a medical defence organisation. We believe prevention is better than cure, so we are more than a last line of defence. Not only do we provide the best defence should you need it, we'll also ensure you have the tools and skills to avoid risks in the first place.

Choose a lifetime of protection. Staying with us when you qualify, and throughout your career, we'll support you every step of the way, with tailored workshops, guidance and advice. However, even the most experienced doctors can find themselves on the receiving end of a complaint, claim or GMC investigation, and it's essential that you have appropriate protection in place, as NHS indemnity is not enough. When that happens, our expert team is here with access to indemnity, world class defence and more.

FREE membership gives you a range of great benefits:
- E-learning modules and OSCE revision resources for your exams
- Exclusive discounts, including up to 25% off medical textbooks
- Protection for your elective
- Expert advice from our medicolegal team available 24/7

To get the most out of your FREE MPS student membership:
- ✓ speak to your MPS representative when they are visiting your medical school, to access discounts and offers
- ✓ visit medicalprotection.org/uk to find out more about your membership benefits and free resources
- ✓ log in and register on My MPS, where you can keep your personal details up to date and won't miss out on new resources and important membership notifications.

How to use this book

The systems chapters

Please note that these chapters are not included in the special MPS edition. Each system chapter covers applied anatomy, history, examination, and the presentation of common and important disorders (available in the main edition from OUP: http://ukcatalogue.oup.com). In each chapter, there are suggestions as to what questions to ask and how to proceed depending on the nature of the presenting complaint. These are not exhaustive and are intended as guidance. The history parts of the systems chapters in the main edition are intended to be used in conjunction with Chapter 2 to build a full and thorough history.

Practical procedures

This chapter describes those practical procedures that the junior doctor or senior nurse may be expected to perform. Some should only be performed once you have been trained specifically in the correct technique by a more senior colleague.

Reality versus theory

In describing the practical procedures, we have tried to be 'realistic'. The methods described are the most commonly used across the profession and are aimed at helping the reader perform the procedure correctly and safely within a clinical environment.

There may be slight differences, therefore, between the way that a small number of the procedures are described here and the way that they are taught in a clinical skills laboratory. In addition, local trusts may use different equipment for some procedures. The good practitioner should be flexible and make changes to their routine accordingly.

Data interpretation

A minority of the reference ranges described for some of the biochemical tests in the data interpretation chapter may differ very slightly from those used by your local laboratory—this is dependent on the equipment and techniques used for measurement. Any differences are likely to be very small indeed. If in doubt, check with your local trust.

Contributors to the main edition

Dr A Abhishek
Consultant Rheumatologist,
Cambridge University Hospitals NHS Trust,
Cambridge, UK

Mr Farid Afshar
Specialty Registrar in Ophthalmology,
Severn Deanery, UK

Dr John Blakey
Senior Clinical Lecturer and Honorary Consultant in Respiratory Medicine,
Liverpool School of Tropical Medicine,
University of Liverpool,
Liverpool, UK

Dr Caroline Bodey
Specialist Registrar in Paediatric Neurodisability,
Leeds, UK

Dr Stuart N Cohen
Consultant Dermatologist,
Nottingham University Hospitals NHS Trust,
Nottingham, UK

Dr Richard Fuller
Associate Professor and Honorary Consultant Physician,
Leeds Institute of Medical Education,
University of Leeds,
Leeds, UK

Mr Venki Sundaram
Specialty Registrar in Ophthalmology,
London Deanery,
London, UK

Symbols and abbreviations

↑	increased
↓	decreased
↔	normal
▶	this fact or idea is important
~	approximately
➜	cross-reference
❶	warning
℗	website
ABG	arterial blood gas
ACTH	adrenocorticotrophic hormone
AMTS	Abbreviated Mental Test Score
ANTT	aseptic non-touch technique
APC	argon plasma coagulation
ATLS	advanced trauma life support
AV	atrioventricular
BMI	body mass index
BSL	British Sign Language
CABG	coronary artery bypass graft
CAH	congenital adrenal hyperplasia
CNS	central nervous system
COPD	chronic obstructive pulmonary disease
CP	cerebral palsy
CPAP	continuous positive airways pressure
CSF	cerebrospinal fluid
CT	computed tomography
DKA	diabetic ketoacidosis
DLCO	carbon monoxide diffusion capacity
DVT	deep vein thrombosis
ECG	electrocardiogram
EMR	endoscopic mucosal resection
ETT	exercise tolerance test
EWS	early warning score
FBC	full blood count
FEV_1	forced expiratory volume in first second
FHx	family history
FNA	fine needle aspiration
FVC	forced vital capacity

GA	general anaesthetic
GCS	Glasgow Coma Scale
GFR	glomerular filtration rate
GOJ	gastro-oesophageal junction
GTN	glyceryl trinitrate
Hb	haemoglobin
HHT	hereditary haemorrhagic telangiectasia
HR	heart rate
IBD	inflammatory bowel disease
IJV	internal jugular vein
INR	international normalized ratio
JVP	jugular venous pressure
LDH	lactate dehydrogenase
LMA	laryngeal mask airway
LV	left ventricle
LVH	left ventricular hypertrophy
MCS	microscopy, culture, and sensitivity
MDI	metered dose inhaler
MDT	multi-disciplinary team
MI	myocardial infarction
MRI	magnetic resonance imaging
NSAIDs	non-steroidal anti-inflammatory drugs
NSF	nephrogenic systemic fibrosis
OGD	oesophagogastroduodenoscopy
OTC	over-the-counter
PC	presenting complaint
PCOS	polycystic ovary syndrome
PEFR	peak expiratory flow rate
PMH	past medical history
PSC	primary sclerosing cholangitis
PTH	parathyroid hormone
PTHrP	parathyroid hormone related protein
RBBB	right bundle branch block
RR	respiratory rate
RV	residual volume
SA	sinoatrial
SBAR	situation, background, assessment, recommendation
SBP	spontaneous bacterial peritonitis
SLE	systemic lupus erythematosus
STD	sexually transmitted disease
SVCO	superior vena cava obstruction

TLC	total lung capacity
TOE	trans-oesophageal echo
UV	ultraviolet
VT	ventricular tachycardia

Chapter 1

Communication skills

Introduction

Communication skills are notoriously hard to teach and describe. There are too many possible situations that one might encounter to be able to draw rules or guidelines. In addition, your actions will depend greatly on the personalities present, not least of all your own.

Using this chapter

Throughout this chapter, there is some general advice about communicating in different situations and to different people. We have not provided rules to stick to, but rather tried to give the reader an appreciation of the great many ways the same situation may be tackled.

Ultimately, skill at communication comes from practice and a large amount of common sense.

A huge amount has been written about communication skills in medicine. Most is a mix of accepted protocols and personal opinion—this chapter is no different.

Patient-centred communication

In recent years, there has been a significant change in the way healthcare workers interact with patients. The biomedical model has fallen out of favour. Instead, there is an appreciation that the patient has a unique experience of the illness involving the social, psychological, and behavioural effects of the disease.

The biomedical model
- Doctor is in charge of the consultation.
- Focus is on disease management.

The patient-centred model (see also Box 1.1)
- Power and decision-making is shared.
- Address and treat the whole patient.

Box 1.1 Key points in the patient-centred model
- Explore the disease and the patient's experience of it:
  - Understand the patient's ideas and feelings about the illness
  - Appreciate the impact on the patient's quality of life and psychosocial well-being
  - Understand the patient's expectations of the consultation.
- Understand the whole person:
  - Family
  - Social environment
  - Beliefs.
- Find common ground on management
- Establish the doctor–patient relationship
- Be realistic:
  - Priorities for treatment.
- Resources.

Becoming a good communicator

Learning

As in all aspects of medicine, learning is a lifelong process. One part of this, particularly relevant to communication skills and at the beginning of your career, is watching others.

The student should take every opportunity to observe doctor–patient and other interactions. Look carefully at how patients are treated by staff that you come across and consider every move that is made...is that something that you could try yourself? Would you like to be treated in that way?

You should ask to be present during difficult conversations.

Instead of glazing over during consultations in clinic or on the ward round, you should watch the interaction and consider if the behaviours you see are worth emulating or avoiding. Consider how you might adjust your future behaviour.

'Cherry-pick' the things you like and use them as your own—building up your own repertoire of communication techniques.

Spontaneity versus learnt behaviours

If you watch a good communicator (in any field) you will see them making friendly conversation, spontaneous jokes, and using words and phrases that put people at ease. It seems natural, relaxed, and spontaneous.

Watching that same person interact with someone else can shatter the illusion as you see them using the very same 'spontaneous' jokes and other gambits from their repertoire.

This is one of the keys to good communication—an ability to judge the situation and pull the appropriate phrase, word, or action from your internal catalogue. If done well, it leads to a smooth interaction with no hesitations or misunderstandings. The additional advantage is that your mental processes are free to consider the next move, mull over what has been said, or consider the findings, whilst externally you are partially on 'auto-pilot'.

During physical examination, this is particularly relevant. You should be able to coax the wanted actions from the patient and put them at ease whilst considering the findings and your next step.

It must be stressed that this is *not* the same as lacking concentration—quite the opposite, in fact.

Essential considerations

Attitudes

Patients are entrusting their health and personal information to you—they want someone who is confident, friendly, competent, and above all, is trustworthy. See Box 1.2 for notes on confidentiality.

Personal appearance

First impressions count—and studies have consistently shown that your appearance (clothes, hair, make-up) has a great impact on the patients' opinion of you and their willingness to interact with you. Part of that intangible 'professionalism' comes from your image.

The white coat is no longer part of the medical culture in the UK. National guidance has widely been interpreted as 'bare below the elbow' with no long sleeves or jewellery. This does not mean that you should look scruffy, however. Many hospitals are now adopting uniforms for all their staff which helps solve some potential appearance issues. Fashions in clothing change rapidly but some basic rules still apply:

- Ensure you have a good standard of personal hygiene.
  - Any perfume or deodorant should not be overpowering
  - Many people believe men should be clean-shaven. This is obviously impossible for some religious groups and not a view shared by the authors. Facial hair should, however, be clean and tidy.
- Neutralize any extreme tastes in fashion that you may have.
- Men should usually wear a shirt. If a tie is worn, it should be tucked into the shirt when examining patients.
- Women may wear skirts or trousers but the length of the skirts should not raise any eyebrows.
- The belly should be covered—even during the summer.
- The shoulders, likewise, should usually be covered.
- Shoes should be polished and clean.
- Clean surgical scrubs may be worn if appropriate.
- Hair should be relatively conservatively styled and no hair should be over the face. It is advised to wear long hair tied up.
- Your name badge should be clearly visible—worn at the belt or on a lanyard around the neck is acceptable depending on hospital policy.
  - Note that lanyards should have a safety mechanism which will allow them to break open if pulled hard. Most hospitals supply these—be cautious about using your own lanyard from a shop or conference
  - Wearing a name badge at the belt means people have to look at your crotch – not necessarily ideal!
- Stethoscopes are best carried—worn at the neck is acceptable but a little pretentious, according to some views.
  - Try not to tuck items in your belt—use pockets or belt-holders for mobile phones, keys, and wallets.

▶ Psychiatry, paediatrics, and a handful of other specialties require a different dress code as they deal with patients requiring differing techniques to bond.

Timing

If in a hospital setting, make sure that your discussion is not during an allocated quiet time—or immediately before one is to start! You should also avoid mealtimes or when the patient's long-lost relative has just come to visit.

▶ If taking the patient from the bedside, ask the supervising doctor (if not you) and the nursing staff—and let all concerned know where you have gone in case the patient is needed.

Setting

Students, doctors, and others tend to see patients on busy wards which provide distractions that can break the interaction. Often this is necessary during the course of a busy day. However, if you are intending to discuss a matter of delicacy requiring concentration on both your parts, consider the following conditions:

- The room should be quiet, private, and free from disturbances.
- There should be enough seating for everyone.
- Chairs should be comfortable enough for an extended conversation.
- Arrange the seats close to yours with no intervening tables or other furniture.

Box 1.2 Confidentiality

As a doctor, healthcare worker, or student, you are party to personal and confidential information. There are certain rules that you should abide by and times when confidentiality must or should be broken. The essence for day-to-day practice is:

Never tell anyone about a patient unless it is directly related to their care.

This includes relatives. Withholding information from family can be very difficult at times, particularly if a relative asks you directly about something confidential.

You can reinforce the importance of confidentiality to relatives and visitors. If asked by a relative to speak to them about a patient, you should approach the patient and ask their permission, preferably within view of the relative.

This rule also applies to friends outside of medicine. As doctors and others, we come across many amazing, bizarre, amusing, or uplifting stories on a day-to-day basis but, like any other kind of information, these should not be shared with anyone, however juicy the story is.

If you do intend to use an anecdote for some after-dinner entertainment, at the very least you should ensure that there is nothing in your story that could possibly lead to the identification of the person or persons involved.

Avoid medical jargon

The problem is that medics are so immersed in jargon that it becomes part of their daily speech. The patient may not understand the words or may have a different idea as to the meaning.

Technical words such as 'myocardial infarction' are in obvious need of avoidance or explanation. Consider terms such as 'exacerbate', 'chronic', 'numb', and 'sputum'—these may seem obvious in meaning to you but not to the patient. Be very careful to tease out the exact meaning of any pseudo-medical terms that the patient uses.

You may also think that some terms such as 'angina' and 'migraine' are well known—but these are very often misinterpreted.

Fear-words

There are certain words which immediately generate fear, such as 'cancer' and 'leukaemia'. You should only use these if you are sure that the patient wants to know the full story.

Beware, however, of avoiding these words and causing confusion by not giving the whole story.

You should also be aware of certain words that people will instinctively assume mean something more serious. For example, to most people a 'shadow' on the lung means cancer. Don't then use the word when you are talking about consolidation due to pneumonia!

The importance of silence

In conversations that you may have with friends or colleagues, your aim is to avoid silence using filler noises such as 'um' and 'ah' whilst pausing.

In medical situations, silences should be embraced and used to extract more information from the patient. Use silence to listen.

Practice is needed as the inexperienced may find this uncomfortable. It is often useful, however, to remain silent once the patient has answered your question. You will usually find that they start speaking again—and often impart useful and enlightening facts.

Remember the name

Forgetting someone's name is what we all fear but is easy to disguise by simple avoidance. However, the use of a name will make you seem to be taking a greater interest. It is particularly important that you remember the patient's name when talking to family. Getting the name wrong is embarrassing and seriously undermines their confidence in you.

Aside from actually remembering the name, it is a good idea to have it written down and within sight—either on a piece of paper in your hand or on the desk, or at the head of the patient's bed. To be seen visibly glancing at the name is forgivable.

Standing

Although this might be considered old-fashioned by some younger people, standing is a universal mark of respect. You should always stand when a patient enters a room and take your seat at the same time as them. You should also stand as they leave but, if you have established a good rapport during the consultation, this isn't absolutely necessary.

Greeting

Beware of 'good afternoon' and 'good morning'. These can be inappropriate if you are about to break some bad news or if there is another reason for distress. Consider instead a simple 'hello'.

Shaking hands

A difficult issue which, again, needs to be judged at the time.

Physical contact always seems friendly and warms a person to you—but a hand-shake may be seen as overly formal by some. It may be inappropriate if the patient is unable to reciprocate through paralysis or pain. Perhaps consider using some other form of touch—such as a slight guiding hand on their arm as they enter the room or a brief touch to the forearm.

Remember also that members of some religious groups may be forbidden from touching a member of the opposite sex.

Introductions

This is a potential minefield! You may wish to alter your greeting depending on circumstances—choose terms that suit you.

Title—them

Older patients may prefer to be called Mr or Mrs; younger patients would find it odd. Difficulty arises with females when you don't know their marital status. Some younger or married patients may find the term 'Ms' offensive.

Using the patient's first name may be considered too informal by some—whilst a change to using the family name mid-way through the encounter will seem very abrasive and unfriendly.

There are no rules here and common sense is required to judge the situation at the time. When unsure, the best option is always to ask.

Title—you

The title 'doctor' has always been a status symbol and a badge of authority—within the healthcare professions, at least. Young doctors may be reluctant to part with the title so soon after acquiring it but, in these days when consultations are becoming two-way conversations between equals, should you really introduce yourself as 'Dr'?

Many patients will simply call you 'doctor' and the matter doesn't arise. The authors prefer using first names in most circumstances but some elderly patients prefer—and expect—a certain level of formality so the situation has to be judged at the time.

Introducing yourself by the first name only seems too informal for most medical situations. Some young-looking students and doctors, however, may feel the need to introduce themselves using their title to avoid any misunderstanding of their role—particularly since the demise of the white coat. Perhaps worth considering is a longer introduction using both your names and an explanation along the lines of 'Hello, my name is Jane Smith, I am one of the doctors.'

General principles

Demeanour

Give the patient your full attention. Appear encouraging with a warm, friendly manner. Use appropriate facial expressions—don't look bored!

Define your role

Along with the standard introductions, you should always make it clear who you are and what your role is. You might also wish to say who your seniors are, if appropriate.

Be sure that anyone else in the room has also been introduced by name.

Style of questioning

Open questions versus closed questions

Open questions are those where any answer is possible. These allow the patient to give you the true answer in their own words. Be careful not to lead them with closed questions.

Compare 'How much does it hurt?' to 'Does it hurt a lot?' The former allows the patient to tell you how the pain feels on a wide spectrum of severity, the latter leaves the patient only two options—and will not give a true reflection of the severity.

Multiple choice questions

Often, patients have difficulty with an open question if they are not quite sure what you mean. A question about the character of pain, for example, is rather hard to form and patients will often not know quite what you mean by 'What sort of pain is it?' or 'What does it feel like, exactly?'

In these circumstances, you may wish to give them a few examples—but leave the list open-ended for them to add their own words. You must be very careful *not* to give the answer that you are expecting from them. For example, in a patient who you suspect has angina ('crushing' pain), you could ask, 'What sort of a pain is it…burning, stabbing, aching, for example…?'

Clarifying questions

Use clarifying questions to get the full details, particularly if there are terms used which may have a different meaning to the patient than to you.

Difficult questions

Apologise for potentially offensive, embarrassing, or upsetting questions ('I'm sorry to have you ask you this, but…').

Reflective comments

Use reflective comments to encourage the patient to go on and reassure them that you are following the story.

Staying on topic

You should be forceful but friendly when keeping the patient on the topic you want or moving the patient on to a new topic. Don't be afraid to interrupt them—some patients will talk for hours if you let them!

Eye-contact

▶ Make eye-contact and look at the patient when they are speaking.

Make a note of eye-contact next time you are in conversation with a friend or colleague.

In normal conversations, the speaker usually looks away whilst the listener looks directly at the speaker. The roles then change when the other person starts talking...and so on.

In the medical situation, whilst the patient is speaking, you may be tempted to make notes, read the referral letter, look at a test result, or similar—you should resist and stick to the 'normal' rules of eye-contact.

Adjusting your manner

You would clearly not talk to another doctor as you would someone with no medical knowledge. This is a difficult area, you should try to adjust your manner and speech according to the patient's educational level.

This can be extremely difficult—you should not make assumptions on intellect or understanding based solely on educational history.

A safe approach is to start in a relatively neutral way and then adjust your manner and speech based on what you see and hear in the first minute or two of the interaction—but be alert to whether this is effective and make changes accordingly.

Interruptions

Apologize to the patient if you are interrupted.

Don't take offence or get annoyed

As well as being directly aggressive or offensive, people may be thoughtless in their speech or manner and cause offence when they don't mean to. As a professional, you should rise above this and remember that apparent aggression may be the patient's coping mechanism, born from a feeling of helplessness or frustration—it is not a personal insult or affront.

Cross-cultural communication

Cultural background and tradition may have a large influence on disease management. Beliefs about the origin of disease and prejudices or stigma surrounding the diagnosis can make dealing with the problem challenging.

Be aware of all possible implications of a person's cultural background, both in their understanding of disease, expectations of healthcare, and in other practices that may affect their health.

Above all, be aware of prejudice—yours and theirs.

Body language: an introduction

Body language is rarely given the place it deserves in the teaching of communication skills. There are over 600 muscles in the human body; 90 in the face of which 30 act purely to express emotion. Changes in your position or expression—some obvious, others subtle—can heavily influence the message that you are communicating.

We've all met someone and thought 'I didn't like him' or alternatively 'she seemed trustworthy'. Often these impressions of people are not built on what is said but the manner in which people handle themselves. You subconsciously pick up cues from the other person's body. Being good at using body language means having awareness of how the other person may be viewing you and getting your subconscious actions and expressions under conscious control.

If done well, you can influence the other person's opinion of you, make them more receptive to your message, or add particular emphasis to certain words and phrases.

Touching

Touching is one of the most powerful forms of non-verbal communication and needs to be managed with care.

- *Greeting:* touch is part of greeting rituals in most cultures. It demonstrates that you are not holding a weapon and establishes intimacy.
- *Shaking hands:* there are many variations. The length of the shake and the strength of the grip impart a huge amount of information. For added intimacy and warmth, a double-handed grip can be used. For extra intimacy, one may touch the other's forearm or elbow.*
- *Dominance:* touch is a powerful display of dominance. Touching someone on the back or shoulder demonstrates that you are in charge—this can be countered by mirroring the action back.
- *Sympathy:* the lightest of touches can be very comforting and is appropriate in the medical situation where other touch may be misread as dominance or intimacy (you shouldn't hug a patient that you've only just met!). Display sympathy by a brief touch to the arm or hand.

Open body language

This refers to a cluster of movements concerned with seeming open. The most significant part of this is the act of opening—signalling a change in the way you are feeling. Openness demonstrates that you have nothing to hide and are receptive to the other person. Openness encourages openness.

This can be used to calm an angry situation or when asking about personal information.

The key is to not have your arms or legs crossed in any way.

---

* Watch the first few minutes of the 1998 film 'Primary Colors' which demonstrates the different uses of touch during handshakes.

- *Arms open:* either at your side or held wide. Even better, hold your hands open and face your palms to the other person.
- *Legs open:* this does not mean legs wide but rather not crossed. You may hold them parallel. The feet often point to something of subconscious interest to you—point them at the patient!

Emphasis

You can amplify your spoken words with your body—usually without noticing it. Actions include nodding your head, pointing, or other hand gestures. A gesture may even involve your entire body.

Watch newsreaders—often only their heads are in view so they emphasize with nods and turns of their heads much more than one would during normal conversation.

- *Synchrony:* this is key. Time points of the finger, taps of the hand on the desk, or other actions with the words you wish to emphasize.
- *Precision:* signal that the words currently being spoken are worth paying attention to with delicate, precise movements. You could make an 'O' with your thumb and index finger or hold your hands such that each finger is touching its opposite counterpart—like a splayed prayer position.

Eye level

This is a very powerful tool. In general, the person with their eye level higher is in control of the situation.

You can use this to your advantage. When asking someone personal questions or when you want them to open up, position yourself such that your eyes are below theirs—meaning they have to look down at you slightly. This makes them feel more in control and comfortable.

Likewise, anger often comes from a feeling of lack of control—put the angry person in charge by lowering your eye level—even if that means squatting next to them or sitting when they are standing.

Conversely, you may raise your eye level to take charge of a difficult situation: looking down on someone is intimidating. Stand over a seated person to demonstrate that you are in charge.

Watch and learn

There is much that could be said about body language. You should watch others and yourselves and consider what messages are being portrayed by non-verbal communication.

Stay aware of your own movements and consider purposefully changing what would normally be subconscious actions to add to, or alter, the meaning of your speech.

Interpreters

Official communicators are bound by a code of ethics, impartiality, and confidentiality—friends and relatives are not.

It is often impossible to be sure that a relative is passing on all that is said in the correct way.

Sometimes, the patient's children are used to interpret—this is clearly not advisable for a number of reasons. This not only places too much responsibility on the child but they may not be able to explain difficult concepts. In addition, conversations about sex, death, or other difficult topics may be unsuitable for the child to be party to.

Using an official interpreter

Before you start
- Brief the interpreter on the situation, clarify your role and the work of the department, if necessary.
- Allow the interpreter to introduce themselves to the patient and explain their role.
- Arrange seating so that the patient can see the interpreter and you equally.
- Allow enough time (at least twice as long as normal).

During the exchange
- Speak to the patient, not the interpreter. This may be hard at first, but you should speak to and look at the patient at all times.
- Be patient, some concepts are hard to explain.
- Avoid complex terms and grammar.
- Avoid jargon.
- Avoid slang and colloquialisms which may be hard to interpret correctly.
- Check understanding frequently.

Finishing off
- Check understanding.
- Allow time for questions.
- ▶ If the conversation has been distressing, offer the interpreter support and let their manager know.

Written information
- If interpreting written information, read it out loud. The interpreter may not necessarily be able to translate written language as easily.
- Many departments and charities provide some written information in a variety of languages—some also provide tapes. You should be aware of what your department has to offer.

Communicating with deaf patients

People who are hard of hearing may cope with the problem by using a hearing-aid, lip-reading, or using sign language. Whichever technique is used (if any), some simple rules should always apply:

- Speak clearly but not too slowly.
- Don't repeat a sentence if it is misunderstood—say the same thing in a different way.
- Write things down if necessary.
- Use plain English and avoid waffling.
- Be patient and take the time to communicate properly.
- Check understanding frequently.
- Consider finding an amplifier—many elderly medicine wards will have one available.

Lip-readers

Patients who are able to lip-read do so by looking at the normal movements of your lips and face during speech. Exaggerating movements or speaking loudly will distort these and make it harder for them to understand. In addition to the points already mentioned, when talking to lip-readers:

- Maintain eye-contact.
- Don't shout.
- Speak clearly but not too slowly.
- Do not exaggerate your oral or facial movements.

British Sign Language (BSL)

- It should be appreciated that BSL is not a signed version of English—it is a distinct language with its own grammar and syntax.
- For BSL users, English is a 2nd or 3rd language so using a pen and paper may not be effective or safe for discussing complex topics or gaining consent.
- Seek an official BSL interpreter, if possible, and follow the rules on working with interpreters.

Telephone communication

The essential rule of confidentiality is that you must not impart personal information to anyone without the express permission of the patient concerned—except in a few specific circumstances.

- You must not give out any confidential information over the telephone as you cannot be sure of the identity of the caller. All communication should be done face-to-face. This may cause difficulty if a relative calls to ask about the patient, but you should remain strict.
- If telephone communication is essential but you are in doubt as to the caller's identity, you may wish to take their number and call them back.

SBAR

SBAR was created as an easy to remember mechanism to frame conversations and install some uniformity into telephone communication, particularly those requiring a clinician's immediate attention and action. There are 4 sections to help you order the information with the right level of detail and reduce repetition.

S: Situation
- Identify yourself (name and designation) and where you are calling from.
- Identify the patient by name and the reason you are calling.
- Describe your concern in one sentence.

Include vital signs where appropriate.

B: Background
- State the admission diagnosis and date.
- Explain the background to the current problem.
- Describe any relevant treatment so far.

You should have collected information from the patient's charts, notes, and drug card and have this at your fingertips. Include current medication, allergies, pertinent laboratory results, and other diagnostic tests.

A: Assessment
- State your assessment of the patient including vital signs, early warning score (EWS), if relevant, and your overall clinical impression and concerns.

You should have considered what might be the underlying reason for the patient's current condition.

R: Recommendation
- 'I think the problem is . . .'.
- Explain what you need and the time-frame in which you need it.
- Make suggestions and clarify expectations.
- 'Is there anything else I should do?'
- ▶ Record the name and contact details of the person you have been speaking to.
- ▶ Record the details of the conversation in the patient's notes.

Other specific situations

Talking about sex

This is a cause of considerable embarrassment for the patient and for the inexperienced professional. Sexual questions are usually inappropriate to be overheard by friends or relatives—so ask them to leave. Your aim is to put the patient at ease and make their responses more forthcoming.

- The key is to ask direct, clear questions and show no embarrassment yourself.
- You should maintain eye-contact.
- You should also show no surprise whatsoever—even if the sexual practices described differ from your own or those that you would consider acceptable.
- Try to become au fait with sexual slang and sexual practices which you might not be familiar with previously.
  - A failure to understand slang may lead to an immediate barrier in the consultation.
- In general, you should not use slang terms first. You may wish to consider mirroring the patient's speech as you continue the conversation.

Angry patients

Use body language to take charge of the situation without appearing aggressive. Throughout the exchange, you should remain polite, avoiding confrontation, and resist becoming angry yourself.

- Look to your own safety first.
- Calm the situation then establish the facts of the case. Anger is often secondary to some other emotion such as loss, fear, or guilt.
- Acknowledge their emotions.
  - 'I can see this has made you angry'
  - 'It's understandable that you should feel like this.'
- Steer the conversation away from the area of unhappiness towards the positive and plans to move the situation forward.
- Don't incriminate colleagues—the patients may remember your throw-away comments which could come back to haunt you. Avoid remarks like 'he shouldn't have done that'.
- Emphasize any grounds for optimism, or plans for resolving the situation and putting things right.

Breaking bad news

Breaking bad news is feared by students and, indeed, no-one likes doing it. However, knowing that you have broken difficult news in a sensitive way and that you have helped the patient through a terrible experience can be one of the most uplifting aspects of working in healthcare.

Before you start
- Confirm all the information for yourself and ensure that you have all the information to hand, if necessary.
- Speak to the nursing staff to get background information on what the patient knows, their fears, and details of the relationship with any family or friends who may be present.

Choose the right place
- Pick a quiet, private room where you won't be disturbed.
- Ensure there is no intervening desk or other piece of furniture.
- Arrange the chairs so that everyone can be seen equally.
- Hand your bleep/mobile phone to a colleague.

Ensure the right people are present
- Invite a member of the nursing staff to join you—particularly if they have already established a relationship with the patient.
  - Remember, it is usually the nursing staff that will be dealing with the patient and relatives when you have left so they need to know exactly what was said.
- Would the patient like anyone present?

Establish previous knowledge
It is essential to understand what the patient already knows. The situation is very different in the case of a patient who knows that you have been looking for cancer to one who thinks their cough is due to a cold.

How much do they want to know?
This is key! Before you consider breaking bad news, you have to discover if the patient actually wants to hear it.
- Ask an open question such as:
  - 'What do you know so far?'
  - 'What have the other doctors/nurses told you?'
- You can also ask directly if they want to hear bad news. Say:
  - 'Are you the sort of person who likes to know all the available facts and details or would you rather a short version?'

Honesty, above all else
- Above all, you should be honest at all times. Never guess or lie.
- The patient may break your pre-prepared flow of information requiring you to think on your feet. Sometimes you simply can't stick to the rules above. If asked a direct question, you must be honest and straightforward.

Warning shots

You should break the news step-wise, delivering multiple 'warning shots'. This gives the patient a chance to stop you if they've heard enough, or to ask for more information. Keep your sentences short, clear, and simple.

You could start by saying that the test results show things are more 'serious' than first thought and wait to see their reaction. If they ask what you mean, you can tell them more, and so on.

▶ Inexperienced practitioners sometimes feel that they 'ought' to tell the patient the full story but they must understand that many people would much rather not hear the words said aloud—this is their coping strategy and must be respected.

Allow time for information to sink in

You should allow time for each piece of information to sink in, ensure that the patient understands all that has been said, and repeat any important information.

Remember also that patients will not be able to remember the exact details of what you have said—you may need to reschedule at a later time to talk about treatment options or prognosis.

Don't rush to the positive

When told of bad news, the patient needs a few moments to let the information sink in. Wait in silence for the patient to speak next.

The patient may break down in tears—in which case they should be offered tissues and the support of relatives, if nearby.

If emotionally distressed, the patient will not be receptive to what you say next—you may want to give them some time alone with a relative or nurse before you continue to talk about prognosis or treatment options.

Above all, you should not give false hope. The moment after the bad news has been broken is uncomfortable and you must fight the instinctive move to the positive with 'there are things we can do', 'on the plus side...', 'the good news is...', or similar.

Questions about time

'How long have I got?' is one of the most common questions to be asked—and the hardest to answer.

- As always, don't guess and don't lie.
- It's often impossible to estimate and is perfectly acceptable to say so. Giving a figure will almost always lead to you being wrong.
- Explain that it is impossible to judge and ask if there is any date in particular that they don't want to miss—perhaps they want to experience Christmas or a relative's birthday.

Ending the conversation

Summarize the information given, check their understanding, repeat any information as necessary, allow time for questions, and make arrangements for a follow-up appointment or a further opportunity to ask questions again.

Obviously, you shouldn't make promises that you can't keep. Don't offer to come back that afternoon if you're going to be in clinic!

Law, ethics, and consent

No discussion of communication skills would be complete without mention of confidentiality, capacity, and consent. It is also worth knowing the four bioethical principles about which much has been written elsewhere.

Four bioethical principles

- *Autonomy:* a respect for the individual and their ability to make decisions regarding their own health.
- *Beneficence:* acting to the benefit of patients.
- *Non-maleficence:* acting to prevent harm to the patient.
- *Justice:* 'fairness' to the patient and the wider community when considering the consequences of an action.

Confidentiality

Confidentiality is closely linked to the ethical principles described above. Maintaining a secret record of personal information shows respect for the individual's autonomy and their right to control their own information. There is also an element of beneficence where releasing the protected information may cause harm.

Breaking confidentiality

The rules surrounding the maintenance of confidentiality have been mentioned. There are a number of circumstances where confidentiality can, or must, be broken. The exact advice varies slightly between different bodies. See the links under 'further reading'. In general, confidentiality may be broken in the following situations:

- With the consent of the individual concerned.
- If disclosure is in the patient's interest but consent cannot be gained.
- If required by law.
- When there is a statutory duty such as reporting of births, deaths, and abortions and in cases of certain communicable diseases.
- If it is overwhelmingly in the public interest.
- If it is necessary for national security or where prevention or detection of a crime may be prejudiced or delayed.
- In certain situations related to medical research.

Consent and capacity

There are three main components to valid consent. To be competent (or have capacity) to give consent, the patient:

- Must understand the information that has been given.
- Must believe that information.
- Must be able to retain and weigh-up the information.

In addition, for consent to be valid, the patient must be free from any kind of duress.

▶ It should be noted that an assessment of capacity is valid for the specific decision in hand. It is not an all-or-nothing phenomenon—you cannot either have 'capacity' or not. The assessment regarding competence must be made for each new decision faced.

Young people and capacity
- All persons aged 18 and over are considered to be a competent adult unless there is evidence to the contrary.
- People aged between 16 and 18 are treated as adults (Family Law Reform Act 1969). However, the refusal of a treatment can be overridden by someone with parental responsibility or the courts.
- Children of 16 and younger are considered competent to give consent if they meet the three conditions mentioned previously. Their decisions can be, however, overridden by the courts or people with parental responsibility.

Gillick competence
In 1985, the well-known Gillick case was considered by the House of Lords and from this two principles (often known as the Fraser Guidelines) were established:
- A parent's right to consent to treatment on behalf of the child finishes when the child has sufficient understanding to give consent themselves (when they become 'Gillick competent').
- The decision as to whether the child is Gillick competent rests with the treating doctor.

Powers of attorney
People lacking mental capacity may need someone to manage their legal, financial, and health affairs. This is done through power of attorney as laid out in the Mental Capacity Act 2005.

Enduring powers of attorney (EPA)
Before 2007, people could grant EPA so a trusted person could manage their finances. Those with EPA do not have the right to make other decisions on a person's behalf.

Lasting powers of attorney (LPA)
Property and affairs LPA
Those with property and affairs LPA can make decisions regarding paying bills, collecting income and benefits, and selling property, subject to any restrictions or conditions the patient may have included.

Personal welfare LPA
This allows the 'attorney' to make decisions relating to living situation and other personal care. They can also make medical decisions *if this power has been expressly given in the LPA.*

Further reading
There are many other complex topics in this area and the law varies between countries and even between regions within the UK. We suggest the following as a good start:
- The British Medical Association: ℘ http://www.bma.org.uk
- The Medical Defence Union: ℘ http://www.the-mdu.com
- The Medical Protection Society: ℘ http://www.medicalprotection.org
- The UK Ministry of Justice: ℘ http://www.justice.gov.uk/
- The UK Department of Health: ℘ http://www.dh.gov.uk

The history

Using this book

This book is divided into chapters by organ system. In each chapter, there are suggestions as to how to proceed depending on the nature of the presenting complaint and notes on what you should especially ask about under each of the standard headings. These are not exhaustive and are intended as guidance to supplement a thorough history.

History taking

The history is a patient's account of their illness together with other relevant information that you have gleaned from them. Like all things in medicine, there is a tried and tested standard sequence which you should stick to and is used by all practitioners.

It is good practice to make quick notes whilst talking to the patient that you can use to write a thorough history afterwards—don't document every word they say as this breaks your interaction!

By the end of the history taking, you should have a good idea as to a diagnosis or have several differential diagnoses in mind. The examination is your chance to confirm or refute these by gaining more information.

History taking is not a passive process. You need to keep your wits about you and gently guide the patient into giving you relevant information using all the communication skills described in ➲ Chapter 1.

You should break the history down into headings and record it in the notes in this order—many people prefer to use the standard abbreviations (shown in Box 2.1) instead of writing out the heading in full.

Box 2.1 The standard history framework
- Presenting complaint (PC)
- History of presenting complaint (HPC)
- Past medical history (PMH)
- Drug history (DHx)
- Allergies/reactions
- Alcohol
- Smoking
- Family history (FHx)
- Social history (SHx)
- Systematic enquiry.

The outline in Box 2.1 is the authors' favoured method—slight variations exist. Remember to record the history thoroughly (see Box 2.2). See also notes on collateral histories in Box 2.3.

▶ Many people will put 'smoking' and 'alcohol' as part of the 'social history'. We feel that as these can have such an important impact on health they deserve their own spot and are more than simply 'what the patient does in their spare time'.

It is good practice in medicine to watch what other practitioners do and adapt the parts that you feel are done well to your own style, making them part of your own routine.

Box 2.2 Recording the history

- Documentation is a vital part of all medical interactions
- The history should be recorded in the patient's notes
- Remember, if it isn't written down, it didn't happen!

Box 2.3 Collateral histories

There are many situations when the patient may be unable to give a history (e.g. they are unconscious, delirious, demented, dysphasic, etc.). In these situations, you should make an effort to speak to all those who can help you fill in the gaps—not only regarding what happened to bring the patient to your attention now, but also regarding their usual medication, functional state, living arrangements, and so on.

When taking a history from a source other than the patient, be sure to document clearly that this is the case and why the patient is unable to speak for themselves.

Useful sources of information include:

- Relatives/cohabitants
- Close friends/room-mates
- The GP or other members of the primary care team
- The pharmacist
- The warden (if in sheltered accommodation)
- The staff at the nursing or residential home
- Anyone who witnessed the event.

Presenting complaint (PC)

- This is the patient's chief symptom(s) in their own words and should be no more than a single sentence.
  - ▶ Remember, this is the problem in the patient's words. 'Haemoptysis' is rarely a presenting complaint but 'coughing up blood' may well be.
- If the patient has several symptoms, present them as a list which you can expand on later in the history.
- Ask the patient an open question such as 'What's the problem?' or 'What made you come to the doctor?' Each practitioner will have their own style. You should choose a phrase that suits you and your manner (one of the authors favours 'tell me the story' after a brief introduction).
  - ❶ The question 'what brought you here?' usually brings the response 'an ambulance' or 'the taxi'—each patient under the impression that they are the first to crack this show-stopper of a joke. This is, therefore, best avoided.

History of the presenting complaint (HPC)

Here, you ask about and document the details of the presenting complaint. By the end of this, you should have a clear idea about the nature of the problem along with exactly how and when it started, how the problem has progressed over time, and what impact it has had on the patient in terms of their general physical health, psychology, social, and working lives.

This is best tackled in two phases:

First, ask an open question and allow the patient to talk through what has happened for about 2 minutes. Don't interrupt! Encourage the patient with non-verbal responses and make discreet notes. This also allows you to make an initial assessment of the patient in terms of education level, personality, and anxiety. Using this information, you can adjust your responses and interaction. It should also become clear to you exactly what symptom the patient is most concerned about.

In the second phase, you should revisit the whole story asking more detailed questions. It may be useful to say 'I'd just like to go through the story again, clarifying some details'. This is your chance to verify time-lines and the relationship of one symptom to another. You should also be careful to clarify pseudo-medical terms (exactly what does the patient mean by 'vertigo', 'flu', or 'rheumatism'?). Remember, this should feel like a conversation, not an interrogation!

▶ The standard features that should be determined for any symptom are shown in Box 2.4; the additional features regarding 'pain' are in Box 2.5.

See Box 2.6 for notes on long-standing symptoms.

At the end of the history of presenting complaint, you should have established a *problem list*. You should run through this with the patient, summarizing what you have been told and ask them if you have the information *correct* and if there is *anything further* that they would like to share with you.

Box 2.4 For each symptom, determine:

- The exact nature of the symptom
- The onset:
  - The date it began
  - How it began (e.g. suddenly, gradually—over how long?)
  - If long-standing, why is the patient seeking help now?
- Periodicity and frequency:
  - Is the symptom constant or intermittent?
  - How long does it last each time?
  - What is the exact manner in which it comes and goes?
- Change over time:
  - Is it improving or deteriorating?
- Exacerbating factors:
  - What makes the symptom worse?
- Relieving factors:
  - What makes the symptom better?
- Associated symptoms.

Box 2.5 SOCRATES

The questions to ask about the characteristics of pain can be remembered with the mnemonic 'SOCRATES':

- S: Site (where is the pain worse? Ask the patient to point to the site with *one finger*)
- O: Onset (how did it come on? Over how long?)
- C: Character (i.e. 'dull', 'aching', 'stabbing', 'burning', etc.)
- R: Radiation (does the pain move or spread to elsewhere?)
- A: Associated symptoms (e.g. nausea, dyspepsia, shortness of breath)
- T: Timing (duration, course, pattern)
- E: Exacerbating and relieving factors
- S: Severity (scored out of 10, with '10' as the worst pain imaginable).

Box 2.6 Long-standing problems

If the symptom is long-standing, ask why the patient is seeking help now. Has anything changed? It is often useful to ask when the patient was last well. This helps focus their minds on the start of the problem which may seem distant and less important to them.

Past medical history (PMH)

Some aspects of the patient's past illnesses or diagnoses may have already been covered. Here, you should obtain detailed information about past illness and surgical procedures.

Ask if they're 'under the doctor for anything else' or have ever been to hospital before. Ensure you get dates and location for each event. There are some conditions which you should specifically ask patients about and these are shown in Box 2.7; see also the notes in Box 2.8.

For each condition, ask:
- When was it diagnosed?
- How was it diagnosed?
- How has it been treated?

For operations, ask about any previous anaesthetic problems.

🚹 Ask also about immunizations and company/insurance medicals.

Box 2.7 PMH – ask specifically about:
- Diabetes
- Rheumatic fever
- Jaundice
- Hypercholesterolaemia
- Hypertension
- Angina
- Myocardial infarction
- Stroke or TIA
- Asthma
- TB
- Epilepsy
- Anaesthetic problems
- Blood transfusions.

Box 2.8 Don't take anything for granted!
- For each condition that the patient reports having, ask exactly how it was diagnosed (where? by whom?) and how it has been treated since
- For example, if the patient reports 'asthma', ask who made the diagnosis, when the diagnosis was made, if they have ever had lung function tests, if they have ever seen a chest physician at a hospital, if they are taking any inhalers
- Occasionally, the patient will give a long-standing symptom a medical name which can be very confusing. In this example, the patient's 'asthma' could be how they refer to their wheeze which is, in fact, due to congestive cardiac failure.

Drug history (DHx)

Here, you should list all the medications the patient is taking, including the dose, duration, and frequency of each prescription along with any significant side effects. If the patient is unsure, you should confirm with the GP or pharmacy. You should make a special note of any drugs that have been started or stopped recently.

You should also ask about compliance/adherence—does the patient know what dose they take? Do they ever miss doses? If they are not taking the medication—what's the reason? Do they have any compliance/adherence aids such as a pre-packaged weekly supply?

The patient may not consider some medications to be 'drugs' so specific questioning is required. Don't forget to ask about:

- Eye drops.
- Inhalers.
- Sleeping pills.
- Oral contraception.
- Over-the-counter drugs (bought at a pharmacy), vitamin supplements.
- Herbal remedies.
- 'Illicit' or 'recreational' drug use (record exactly what type of drug, route of administration, site, frequency of use, shared needles).

Allergies and reactions

This should be documented separately from the 'drug history' due to its importance.

Ask if the patient has any allergies or 'is allergic to anything' if they are unfamiliar with the term. Be sure to probe carefully as people will often tell you about their hay fever and forget about the rash they had when they took penicillin. Ask specifically if they have had any 'reactions' to drugs or medication.

▶ If an allergy is reported, you should obtain the exact nature of the event and decide if the patient is describing a true allergy, an intolerance, or simply an unpleasant side effect.

▶ All true allergies should be clearly recorded in the patient's case notes and drug chart.

Alcohol

Attempt to quantify, as accurately as you can, the amount and type of alcohol consumed daily/per week—and also establish if the consumption is spread evenly over the week or concentrated into a shorter period.

In the UK, alcohol is quantified in 'units' (1 unit = 10ml of alcohol).

In many European countries, and the US, alcohol is quantified as 'standard drinks'. In the US, a 'standard drink' contains 0.54 ounces of alcohol which is about 1.5 UK 'units'.

Units can be calculated as in Box 2.9 and Box 2.10.

If there is a suspicion of excess alcohol consumption, you may wish to use the quick 'CAGE and 'FAST' questionnaires shown in Boxes 2.11 and 2.12.

Recommended weekly alcohol consumption

- The Royal College of Physicians advises no more than 21 units per week for men and 14 units per week for women.
- The UK Department for Health advises alcohol consumption should not regularly exceed 3–4 units daily for men and 2–3 units daily for women.
- Both men and women should have at least 2 alcohol-free days per week.

Box 2.9 Calculating units
- You can work out how many units there are in any drink by multiplying the total volume of a drink (in ml) by its % alcohol by volume (ABV) or 'strength'. Divide the result by 1000
  - (Strength x volume)/1000
- Example:
  - 1 pint (568ml) of strong lager (ABV 5.2%)
  - = (5.2 x 568)/1000
  - = 2.95 units.

Box 2.10 Unit content of common drinks
- 1 unit = ½ pint of normal beer, single spirit shot
- 1.5 units = small glass of wine (125ml), bottle of alcopop
- 2 units = large bottle/can/pint normal beer, ½ pint of strong beer, medium glass of wine (175ml)
- 3 units = large bottle/can strong beer, large glass of wine (250ml)
- 9 units = bottle of wine
- 30 units = bottle of spirits.

Box 2.11 CAGE questionnaire

A positive response to any of the four questions may indicate someone at risk of alcohol abuse. A positive answer to two or more questions makes the presence of alcohol dependency likely.

- C: Have you ever felt that you should <u>C</u>ut down your drinking?
- A: Have you ever become <u>A</u>ngry when someone suggested that you should cut down?
- G: Do you ever feel <u>G</u>uilty about your drinking?
- E: Do you ever need an '<u>E</u>ye-opener' in the morning to steady your nerves or get rid of a hangover?

Box 2.12 FAST questionnaire (Fast Alcohol Screening Test)

- This questionnaire is used to identify hazardous drinking
- '1 drink' is defined as '1 unit' or ½ pint of beer, 1 glass of wine or 1 single spirit:

1. Men: How often do you have 8 or more drinks on one occasion?
1. Women: How often do you have 6 or more drinks on one occasion?

Never   Less than monthly   Monthly   Weekly   Daily

2. How often during the last year have you been unable to remember what happened the night before because you had been drinking?

Never   Less than monthly   Monthly   Weekly   Daily

3. How often during the last year have you failed to do what was normally expected of you because of drink?

Never   Less than monthly   Monthly   Weekly   Daily

4. In the last year, has a relative, or friend, or doctor, or other health worker been concerned about your drinking or suggested you cut down?

No   Yes, once   Yes, more than once

Scoring
- Question 1: never = not misusing alcohol; weekly/ daily = hazardous or harmful drinking. If other responses, go on to question 2
- Questions 1, 2, and 3: score each answer as 0, 1, 2, 3, 4 with never as 0 and daily as 4
- Question 4: no = 0; yes, once = 2; yes, more than once = 4
- Maximum score = 16.

The patient is misusing alcohol if the total score is more than 3.

Smoking

- Attempt to quantify the habit in 'pack-years'. 1 pack-year is 20 cigarettes per day for one year (e.g. 40/day for 1 year = 2 pack-years; 10/day for 2 years = 1 pack-year).
  - An alternative calculation which gets you the same result: (no. of cigarettes smoked per day x number of years)/20.
- Ask about previous smoking as many will call themselves non-smokers if they gave up yesterday or even on their way to the hospital or clinic. See Box 2.13 for notes on quantification.
- Remember to ask about passive smoking.
  - ❶ Be aware of cultural issues—smoking is forbidden for Sikhs, for example, and they may take offence at the suggestion.

Health problems related to tobacco

Cardiovascular
- Coronary heart disease.
- Peripheral vascular disease.
- Abdominal aortic aneurysm.

Respiratory
- COPD.
- Bronchitis.
- Pneumonia.

Neurological
- Cerebrovascular disease.

Sexual
- Erectile and ejaculatory dysfunction.

Neoplasias
- Oral cavity.
- Laryngeal.
- Pharyngeal.
- Bronchial/lung.
- Oesophageal.
- Gastric.
- Pancreatic.
- Renal.
- Cystic.
- Cervical.
- Acute myeloid leukaemia.

Other
- Infertility.
- Pre-term delivery.
- Still-birth.
- Low birth weight.
- Sudden infant death syndrome.

Some conditions where smoking can worsen symptoms

- Asthma.
- Chest infections including tuberculosis.
- Chronic rhinitis.
- Diabetic retinopathy.
- Optic neuritis.
- Hyperthyroidism.
- Multiple sclerosis.
- Crohn's disease.

Some conditions which smoking increases the risk of

- Dementia.
- Optic neuropathy.
- Cataracts.
- Macular degeneration.
- Pulmonary fibrosis.
- Psoriasis.
- Gum disease.
- Tooth loss.
- Osteoporosis.
- Raynaud's phenomenon.

Box 2.13 Haggling and the art of quantification

Smoking and alcohol histories are notoriously unreliable—alcohol especially so. The patient may be trying to please you or feel embarrassed about openly admitting their true consumption.

Gaining an accurate account of consumption can sometimes feel like haggling. There are two steps in this process.

Firstly, appear non-judgemental and resist acting surprised *in any way*, even in the face of liquor or tobacco consumption that you may consider excessive and unwise.

Secondly, if the patient remains reticent ('I smoke a few'), suggest a number—but start very high ('shall we say 60 a day?') and the patient will usually give you a number nearer the true amount ('oh no, more like 20'). If you were to start low, the same patient may only admit to half that.

Family history (FHx)

The FHx details:
- The make up of the current family, including the age and gender of parents, siblings, children, and extended family as relevant.
- The health of the family.

You should ask about any diagnosed conditions in other living family members. You should also document the age of death and cause of death for all deceased first-degree relatives and other family members if you feel it is appropriate.

It is worth noting that whilst many conditions run in families, some are due to a single gene disorder. If this is the case (such as Huntington's disease and cystic fibrosis) you should go back several generations for details of consanguinity and racial origins.

It may help to draw a family tree as shown in Box 2.14. These are particularly useful in paediatric assessments.

Social history (SHx)

This is your chance to document the details of the patient's personal life which are relevant to the working diagnosis, the patient's general well-being, and recovery/convalescence. It will help to understand the impact of the illness on the patient's functional status.

This is a vital part of the history but sadly, perhaps because it comes at the end, it is often given only brief attention. The disease, and indeed the patient, do not exist in a vacuum but are part of a community which they interact with and contribute to. Without these details, it is impossible to take an holistic approach to the patient's well-being.

Establish:
- Marital status, sexual orientation.
- Occupation (or previous occupations if retired).
  - You should establish the exact nature of the job if it is unclear—does it involve sitting at a desk, carrying heavy loads, travelling?
- Other people who live at the same address.
- The type of accommodation (e.g. house, flat—and on what floor).
- Does the patient own their accommodation or rent it?
- Are there any stairs? How many?
- Does the patient have any aids or adaptations in their house (e.g. rails near the bath, stairlift)?
- Does the patient use any walking aids (e.g. stick, frame, scooter)?
- Does the patient receive any help day-to-day?
  - Who from (e.g. family, friends, social services)?
  - Who does the laundry, cleaning, cooking, and shopping?
- Does the patient have relatives living nearby?
- What hobbies does the patient have?
- Does the patient own any pets?
- Has the patient been abroad recently or spent any time abroad in the past (countries visited, travel vaccination, malaria prophylaxis)?
- Does the patient drive?

Box 2.14 Family trees

Conventionally, males are represented by a square (□) and females by a circle (○). The patient that you are talking to is called the *propositus* and is indicated by a small arrow (↗).

Horizontal lines represent marriages or relationships resulting in a child. Vertical lines descend from these, connecting to a horizontal line from which the children 'hang'. You can add ages and causes of death.

Family members who have died are represented by a diagonal line through their circle or square (⌀, ⌀) and those with the condition of interest are represented by shaded shapes (●, ■).

See Figs 2.1 and 2.2 for examples of family trees.

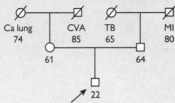

Fig. 2.1 Our patient is an only child and has no children, his parents are alive but all his grandparents have died of different causes.

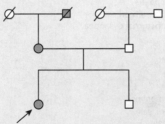

Fig. 2.2 Our patient suffers from colon cancer and has no children. She has a brother who is well. Her parents are both alive and her mother also has colon cancer. Of her grandparents, only her paternal grandfather is alive. Her maternal grandfather died of colon cancer.

Systematic enquiry (SE)

After talking about the presenting complaint, you should perform a brief screen of the other bodily systems.

This often proves to be more important than you expect, finding symptoms that the patient had forgotten about or identifying secondary, unrelated, problems that can be addressed.

The questions asked will depend on the discussion that has gone before. If you have discussed chest pain in the history of presenting complaint, there is no need to ask about it again.

General symptoms
- Change in appetite (loss or gain).
- Fever.
- Lethargy.
- Malaise.

Respiratory symptoms
- Cough.
- Sputum.
- Haemoptysis.
- Shortness of breath.
- Wheeze.
- Chest pain.

Cardiovascular symptoms
- Shortness of breath on exertion.
- Paroxysmal nocturnal dyspnoea.
- Chest pain.
- Palpitations.
- Ankle swelling.
- Orthopnoea.
- Claudication.

Gastrointestinal symptoms
- Weight loss or gain.
- Abdominal pain.
- Indigestion.
- Dysphagia.
- Odynophagia.
- Nausea.
- Vomiting.
- Change in bowel habit, diarrhoea, constipation.
- PR blood loss.

Genitourinary symptoms
- Urinary frequency.
- Polyuria.
- Dysuria.
- Haematuria.
- Nocturia.

Neurological symptoms
- Headaches.
- Dizziness.
- Tingling.
- Weakness.
- Tremor.
- Fits, faints, 'funny turns'.
- Black-outs.
- Sphincter disturbance.

Endocrine symptoms
- Heat or cold intolerance.
- Neck swelling (thyroid).
- Menstrual disturbance.
- Erectile dysfunction.
- Increased thirst.
- Sweating, flushing.
- Hirsutism.
- Muscle weakness.

Locomotor symptoms
- Aches, pains.
- Stiffness.
- Swelling.

Skin symptoms
- Lumps/bumps.
- Ulcers.
- Rashes.
- Other lesions (e.g. skin colour or texture change).
- Itch.

Sexual history

A detailed sexual history does not form part of the standard routine. However, if the patient complains of genitourinary symptoms, a full and thorough sexual history should be obtained.

This can be awkward for both the patient and the history taker. It should be undertaken in a sensitive, confident, and confidential manner. Before the discussion takes place, the patient should be reassured about the levels of privacy and confidentiality and that they are free to openly discuss their sexual life and habits.

Make no assumptions, remain professional, and try to use the patient's own words and language. Beware of cultural and religious differences surrounding both sex and talking about it.

You should approach a sexual history in a structured way.

Sexual activity

This should include an assessment of the risk of acquiring a sexually transmitted disease (STD).

You need to determine the number and gender of the patient's sexual partners, what their risk of having an STD is and what precautions (if any) were taken. Try asking the following questions:

- Do you have sex with men, women, or both?
- In the past 2 months, how many people have you had sex with?
- When did you last have sexual intercourse?
- Was it with a man or a woman?
- Were they a casual or regular partner?
- Where were they from?
- Do they use injected drugs?
- Do they have any history of STDs?
- How many other partners do you think they've had recently?
- In what country did you have sex?
- What kind of sex did you take part in (e.g. vaginal, anal, oral)?
- For each type of sex…did you use a condom?
- Does your partner have any symptoms?
- Have you had any other partners in the last 6 weeks?
  - If so, repeat the questions for each partner.

Previous history

You also need to establish the history of STDs for the patient.

- Have you had any other STDs?
- Have you ever had a sexual check-up?
- Have you ever been tested for HIV, hepatitis, or syphilis?
- Have you ever been vaccinated against hepatitis A or B?

Psychological factors

Concerns over loss of libido and sexual functioning may point to a complex psychological cause for the symptoms. Explore this delicately and ask about:

- A history of sexual abuse.
- Problems with the relationship.
- Sexual partners outside the relationship.
- Any other cause for anxiety.
- A history of depression or anxiety.

The elderly patient

Obtaining a history from older people might be regarded as no greater a task than from any patient—however cognitive decline, deafness, acute illness, and the middle of a night shift can make this difficult. Getting to grips with taking a good history from older people is a skill you will find useful in all other situations. Whilst the history is key for making diagnoses, it is an opportunity for so much more—your first interaction with an (older) patient sets important first impressions. A skilful history not only reaps diagnostic rewards, but marks you as a competent doctor who can gain trust, reassure, and communicate well with patients in any challenging situation (see Boxes 2.15 and 2.16 for more).

Box 2.15 Learning to listen

It can be tempting to ask lots of questions to obtain every fact in the history, particularly if you are rushed and faced with a clerking pro forma. Doing this will not only frustrate and offend your patient (because you clearly don't listen), but will also risk you missing important facts.

Instead, learn to stay quiet—and listen in detail to the history of the presenting complaint which may only be 3–4 minutes, but gives your patient a chance to be heard; seemingly irrelevant detail is often useful when patients have the chance to put it in context. It often saves you time, as other key information may emerge straight away and you can better focus the history.

Key points

- *Problem lists:* patients with chronic illness or multiple diagnoses may have more than one strand to their acute presentation. Consider breaking the history of the presenting complaint down into a problem list e.g. (1) worsening heart failure; (2) continence problems; (3) diarrhoea; (4) falls. This can often reveal key interactions between diagnoses you might not have thought about.
- *Drug history:* remember polypharmacy and that patients may not remember all the treatments they take. Be aware that more drugs mean more side effects and less concordance—so ask which are taken and why—(older) people are often quite honest about why they omit tablets. Eye drops, sleeping pills, and laxatives are often regarded as non-medicines by patients, so be thorough and ask separately—and avoid precipitating delirium due to acute withdrawal of benzodiazepines.
- *Past history:* as well as the traditional list of illnesses, remember to ask about recent admissions, whether to hospital or community/ intermediate care facilities. Do they see other disciplines in outpatients?
- *Functional history:* a comprehensive functional history is a cornerstone of your history taking in older people—we make no apologies for reminding you about this throughout this book. Diseases may not be cured or modified, but their key component—the effects on patients

and their lives—might be easily transformed through manipulation of activities of daily living. Remember to ask about formal and informal support for the patient at home—have things resulted in a crisis for the patient because a caring neighbour or friend is unwell? Be polite— and ask tactfully about benefits, including Attendance Allowance— many patients do not realize they might be eligible, so couch your questions with an explanation that advice might be available too.

- *Social history:* is exactly that, and should complement the functional history. Occupation (other than 'retired') can be of value when faced with a new diagnosis of pulmonary fibrosis or bladder cancer and may give your patient a chance to sketch out more about their lives. Enquire about family—don't assume that a relative may be able to undertake more help, as they may live far away; the patient may still have a spouse but be separated. Chat with patients about their daily lives—understanding interests and pursuits can help distract an unwell patient, give hope for the future, and act as a spur for recovery and meaningful rehabilitation. Learn to consider not just the patient and their acute illness, but a wider context that involves home, family, and potential issues such as carer strain.

Box 2.16 A note on narratives

Akin to 'learning to listen' is the recognition that many patients might not deliver their histories in a style that fits the traditional pattern described in this chapter. Pushing (older) patients through histories is not to be recommended. Elders will often discuss events and preferences with a constituted story, and it is important to recognize the value of this. Narrative analysis at its most simple—i.e. your ability to listen and interpret—is a vital skill for all clinicians. Listening to stories allows you to understand patients' preferences, hopes, and fears.

Remember also that older patients often have different views about what they want from their doctors. Their 'agendas' may differ hugely from what you think treatment plans should be, but they may not make their views known through fear of offending you. If you are unsure, always ask—learning to involve your patients in key decisions about their care will make you a better clinician.

Chapter 3

General and endocrine examination

The eye in endocrine disease

Please turn to ➜ Chapter 9 for details of:
- Examination of the fundus.
- Eye signs in thyroid disease.
- The fundus in endocrine disease including diabetic retinopathy.

Approaching the physical examination

General conduct

Medical professionals are in a position of trust. It is generally assumed that you will act with professionalism, integrity, honesty, and with a respect for the dignity and privacy of your patients. In no part of the patient encounter is this more evident than at the physical examination.

People who you may have only just met will take off their clothes and allow you to look at and touch their bodies—something that would be completely unacceptable to many people in any other situation. They will, of course, be more comfortable with this if you have established an appropriate rapport during history taking. However, the communication does not stop at the end of the history. The manner in which you conduct yourself during the examination can make the difference between an effective examination and a formal complaint.

This is not to say that you should shy away from examining for fear of acting inappropriately and causing offence. In particular, you should not avoid examining members of the opposite sex, especially their intimate body parts, as there should be no sexual undertones in the relationship.

Projected confidence will be picked up by the patient, making them more at ease. Constant verbal and non-verbal communication should ensure that no misunderstandings occur. You should ensure that you have a chaperone present—another student, doctor, nurse, or other healthcare professional—whenever you perform any intimate examination. The chaperone should ideally be the same gender as the patient.

The format of the examination

The 'right' approach

One important rule is that you should always stand at the patient's right hand side. It is thought this gives them a feeling of control over the situation (most people are right handed), although there is no hard evidence to this effect. All the standard examination techniques are formulated with this orientation in mind.

The systems examinations

The physical examination can be broken into body systems—and this is the format of this book.

You often need to examine several systems at a time and it is then that you must combine your learnt techniques.

The examination framework

Each system examination is divided into 4 categories:
- Inspection (looking).
- Palpation (feeling).
- Percussion (tapping).
- Auscultation (listening).

In addition, there may be special tests and other added categories—but you will meet these as you go through the book.

First impressions

Diagnosis at first sight

From the first moment you set eyes on the patient, you should be forming impressions of their general state of health. It takes experience and practice to pick up all the possible clues but much can be gained by combining common sense with medical knowledge. Ask yourself:

- Is the patient comfortable or distressed?
- Is the patient well or ill?
- Is there a recognizable syndrome or facies?
- Is the patient well-nourished and hydrated?

Many of these features will be noted subconsciously—but you must make yourself consciously aware of them.

Bedside clues

In a hospital setting, there may be additional clues as to the patient's state of health in the objects around them. In other circumstances, look at objects that they are carrying or are visible in their pockets.

Examples include oxygen tubing, inhalers, GTN spray, insulin injections, glucose meter, or cigarettes.

Vital signs

It may also be appropriate to assess vital signs at an early stage. These usually include:

- Temperature.
- Blood pressure.
- Pulse.
- Oxygen saturation.
- Respiratory rate.
- Blood glucose.

Conscious level

If necessary, a rapid and initial assessment of a patient's conscious level can be made using the AVPU scale or the GCS.

Set-up

Before commencing a formal examination, introduce yourself, explain what you would like to do and obtain verbal consent.

- Ensure that the patient has adequate privacy to undress.
- Make sure that you will not be disturbed.
- Check that the examination couch or bed is draped/covered by a clean sheet or disposable towelling.
- If the patient is accompanied, ask them if they would like their companion(s) to stay in the room.
- Check that any equipment you will require is available (torch, cotton wool, tendon hammer, stethoscope, etc.).
- When ready, the patient should ideally be positioned supine with the head and shoulders raised to ~45°.

Colour

The colour of the patient, or parts of the patient, can give clues to their general state of health and to particular diagnoses. Look especially for evidence of pallor, central and peripheral cyanosis, jaundice, and abnormal skin pigmentation.

Pallor (paleness)

Facial pallor is often a sign of severe anaemia and is especially noticeable on inspecting the palpebral conjunctiva, nail beds, and palmar skin creases.

Ask the patient to look upward and gently draw down their lower eyelid with your thumb—the conjunctiva should be red/pink.

It is, however, an unreliable sign in shocked patients and those with vascular disease since peripheral vasoconstriction or poor blood flow causes skin and conjunctival pallor, even in the absence of blood loss.

Cyanosis

Cyanosis refers to a bluish discoloration of the skin and mucous membranes and is due to the presence of at least 2.5g/dl of deoxygenated haemoglobin in the blood.

Central cyanosis: the tongue appears blue due to an abnormal amount of deoxygenated blood in the arteries. This may develop in any lung disease in which there is a ventilation/perfusion mismatch such as chronic obstructive pulmonary disease ± cor pulmonale and massive pulmonary embolus. It will also occur in right to left cardiac shunts. Finally, polycythaemia and haemoglobinopathies (such as methaemoglobinaemia and sulphaemoglobinaemia) may give the appearance of cyanosis due to abnormal oxygen carriage.

Peripheral cyanosis: a bluish discoloration at the extremities (fingers, toes) only. It is usually due to a ↓ in blood supply or a slowing of the peripheral circulation. The latter commonly arises through exposure to cold, reduced cardiac output, or peripheral vascular disease.

Jaundice

Jaundice (icterus) refers to a yellow pigmentation of those tissues in the body which contain elastin (skin, sclerae, and mucosa) and occurs due to an ↑ in plasma bilirubin (visible at >35micromol/L).

Jaundice is best appreciated in fair-skinned individuals in natural daylight. Expose the sclera by gently holding down the lower lid and asking the patient to look upwards.

▶ Jaundice should not be confused with carotenaemia, which also causes a yellow discoloration of the skin, but the sclerae remain white.

Other abnormalities of coloration

You will meet other distinctive colour patterns through this book, a list here would be lengthy and probably unnecessary. These include the classic slate-grey appearance of haemochromatosis, the silver-grey coloration in argyria (silver poisoning), the ↑ skin-fold pigmentation seen in Addison's disease, and the non-pigmented patches of vitiligo.

Temperature

- Record the patient's temperature using either a mercury or electronic thermometer.
- The recording will depend on the site of measurement.
  - Normal oral temperature is usually considered to be 37°C
  - Rectal temperature is 0.5°C higher
  - Axillary temperature is 0.5°C lower.
- There is also a diurnal variation in body temperature.
  - Peak temperatures occur between 6pm and 10pm
  - Lowest temperatures occur between 2am and 4am.

High temperature

- The febrile pattern of most diseases also follows the diurnal variation described. Sequential recording of temperature may show a variety of patterns which can be helpful in diagnosis.
  - Persistent pyrexia may be a sign of malignant hyperthermia, a drug fever (e.g. halothane, suxamethonium), typhus, or typhoid fever
  - An intermittent pyrexia can be suggestive of lymphomas and pyogenic infections such as miliary TB
  - A relapsing high temperature or Pel–Ebstein fever occasionally occurs in patients with Hodgkin's disease and is characterized by 4–5 days of persistent fever which then returns to baseline before rising again.
- Also note any rigors (uncontrollable shaking) which may accompany high fever and are often considered characteristic of biliary sepsis or pyelonephritis, although can occur in the context of any sepsis.

Low temperature

- Hypothermia is a core (rectal) temperature of <35°C and occurs usually from cold exposure (e.g. near-drowning) or secondary to an impaired level of consciousness (e.g. following excess alcohol or drug overdose) or in the elderly (e.g. myxoedema).
- Patients may be pale with cold, waxy skin and stiff muscles, consciousness is often reduced.
- Patients typically lose consciousness at temperatures <27°C.

Hydration

You may already have obtained clues regarding hydration status from the history. For example, a patient may have been admitted with poor fluid intake and may feel thirsty. Sepsis, bleeding, or bowel obstruction and vomiting can also cause a person to become dehydrated.

Examination

- Begin with looking around the patient for any obvious clues including fluid restriction signs, catheter bag, or nutritional supplements.
- Inspect the face for sunken orbits (moderate–severe dehydration).
- *Mucous membranes:* inspect the tongue and mucous membranes for moisture.
  - Dehydration will cause these surfaces to appear dry.
- *Skin turgor:* assess by gently pinching a fold of skin on the forearm, holding for a few moments, and letting go.
  - If normally hydrated, the skin will promptly return to its original position, whereas in dehydration (reduced skin turgor), the skin takes longer to return to its original state
  - ❗ This sign is unreliable in elderly patients whose skin may have lost its normal elasticity.
- *Capillary refill:* test by raising the patient's thumb to the level of the heart, pressing hard on the pulp for 5 seconds, and then releasing. Measure the time taken for the normal pink colour to return.
  - Normal capillary refill time should be <2 seconds; a prolongation is indicative of a poor blood supply to the peripheries.
- *Pulse rate:* a compensatory tachycardia may occur in dehydration or in fluid overload.
- *Blood pressure:* check lying and standing blood pressure readings and look for a low blood pressure on standing (orthostatic hypotension) which may suggest dehydration.
- *JVP:* Assess the height of the JVP which is one of the most sensitive ways of judging intravascular volume.
  - The JVP is low in dehydration, but raised in fluid overload (e.g. pulmonary oedema).
- *Oedema:* another useful sign of fluid overload (think right heart failure, constrictive pericarditis, hypoalbuminaemia). Remember to test for both ankle and sacral oedema.

Oedema

Oedema refers to fluid accumulation in the tissues, particularly the subcutaneous layer, and implies an imbalance of the Starling forces (↑ intravascular pressure or reduced intravascular oncotic pressure) causing fluid to seep into the interstitial space.

Oedema will occur in hypoproteinaemic states (especially nephrotic syndrome, malnutrition, and malabsorption) and severe cardiac and renal failure.

Other causes of leg swelling are outlined in Box 3.1.

Examination

In ambulant patients, palpate the medial distal shaft of the tibia (the 'bare area') for oedema by gently compressing for up to 10 seconds with the thumb. If the oedema is 'pitting', the skin will show an indentation where pressure was applied which refills slowly.

▶ If oedema is present, note how far it extends proximally. What is the highest point at which you can detect oedema? Peripheral oedema may also involve the anterior abdominal wall and external genitalia.

When lying down, fluid moves to the new dependent area causing a 'sacral pad'. This can be checked for by asking the patient to sit forwards, exposing the lower back and sacral region, and again applying gentle pressure with your fingertips.

Box 3.1 Some causes of leg swelling

Local causes
- Cellulitis (usually unilateral)
- Ruptured Baker's cyst (usually unilateral)
- Occlusion of a large vein—i.e. thrombophlebitis, deep vein thrombosis (DVT), extrinsic venous compression
- Chronic venous insufficiency—pigmentation induration, inflammation, lipodermatosclerosis
- Lipomatosis
- Gastrocnemius rupture—swelling and bruising around the ankle joint and foot.

Systemic causes
- Congestive cardiac failure
- Hypoproteinaemia (nephrotic syndrome, liver cirrhosis, protein-losing enteropathy, kwashiorkor)
- Hypothyroidism
- Hyperthyroidism
- Drugs (e.g. corticosteroids, NSAIDs, vasodilators).

Lymphoedema
- This is non-pitting oedema associated with thickened and indurated skin
- It can be idiopathic or secondary to proximal lymphatic obstruction such as post surgery, metastatic cancer, or chronic infection.

Nutritional status

The nutritional status of the patient may be an important marker of disease and is often overlooked in physical examination.

There are simple clinical measures with can easily be undertaken to assess a patient's overall nutritional status.

General physical appearance

- Note the patient's overall body habitus; are they fat or thin?
- Do they appear to have recently lost or gained weight?
  - Weight loss can lead to muscle wasting seen as skeletal prominence, especially cheek bones, head of humerus, major joints, rib cage, and the bony landmarks of the pelvis.

Body weight and height

All patients should be weighed using accurate scales and have their height recorded (ideally using a stadiometer).

Body mass index

The body mass index (BMI) is a useful estimate of body fatness.

$$BMI = \frac{weight(kg)}{[height(m)]^2}$$

The World Health Organization has classified BMI as follows:

- 19–25 = normal.
- 25–30 = overweight.
- 30–40 = obese.
- >40 = extreme or 'morbid' obesity.

Regional fat distribution

A central distribution of fat (waist:hip circumference ratio of >1.0 in men and >0.9 in women) is associated with higher morbidity and mortality.

Skin fold thickness

Skin fold thickness is another useful method of assessing muscle and fat status and is usually measured at the triceps halfway between the olecranon and acromial processes. This is measured using specialist calipers.

The examiner should pinch a fold of skin and subcutaneous tissue between thumb and first finger and then apply the calipers to the skin fold. Three measurements are normally taken and the average calculated (normal values are 20mm in men and 30mm in women).

Mid-arm circumference

An additional method for estimating body fatness at the bedside is to measure mid-arm muscle circumference.

As with skin fold thickness, use the midpoint between the tip of the olecranon and acromial processes as your standard measurement point.

With the arm in a flexed right-angle position, take 3 tape measurements at this point before calculating the average. Standard age/sex charts are available.

Some conditions associated with malnutrition

- Any very ill patient.
- Malignancy.
- Metabolic disease (e.g. renal failure).
- Gastrointestinal disease (especially small bowel).
- Sepsis.
- Trauma.
- Post-surgery.
- Psychosocial problems (e.g. depression, anorexia nervosa, social isolation).

Some conditions associated with obesity

- Simple obesity ('biopsychosocial').
- Genetic e.g. Prader–Willi, Lawrence–Moon–Biedl syndrome.
- Endocrine (e.g. Cushing's syndrome, hypothyroidism).
- Drug-induced (e.g. corticosteroids).
- Hypothalamic damage due to tumour or trauma.

Lymph nodes

An examination of the lymph nodes forms part of the routine for most body systems. As there is no need to percuss or auscultate, examination involves inspection followed by palpation.

It should be remembered that there are a great many lymph nodes that are not accessible to the examining hand—for example, along the aorta, in the intestinal mesentery, and so on. There are several groups of lymph nodes that are accessible for the purposes of physical examination.

In the head and neck, these are located along the anterior and posterior aspects of the neck and on the underside of the jaw. In the upper limb and trunk, lymph nodes are located in the epitrochlear and axillary regions and in the lower limbs nodes can be examined in the inguinal and popliteal regions.

▶ Remember that the liver and spleen are often enlarged in the presence of generalized lymphadenopathy and these should be examined.

Inspection

Large nodes are often clearly visible on inspection, particularly if the enlargement is asymmetrical. If nodes are infected, the overlying skin may be red and inflamed.

Palpation

Lymph nodes should be palpated using the most sensitive part of your hands—the fingertips.

- *Head and neck (see Fig. 3.1):* the nodes should be palpated with the patient in an upright position and the examiner standing behind—similar to the examination of the thyroid gland.
- *Axillae (see Fig. 3.2):* To examine the nodes at the right axilla:
  - The patient should be sitting comfortably and you should stand at their right-hand side
  - Support their right arm abducted to 90° with your right hand
  - Examine the axilla with your left hand
  - To examine the nodes at the left axilla, perform the opposite manoeuvre.
- *Inguinal (see Fig. 3.3):* with the patient lying supine, palpate their inguinal region along the inguinal ligament—the same position as feeling for a hernia or the femoral pulse.
  - There are 2 chains of superficial inguinal lymph nodes—a horizontal chain which runs just below the inguinal ligament and a vertical chain which runs along the saphenous vein.
- *Epitrochlear nodes:* place the palm of the right hand under the patient's slightly flexed right elbow and feel with your fingers in the groove above and posterior to the medial epicondyle of the humerus.
- *Popliteal:* best examined by passively flexing the knee and exploring the fossa with the fingers of both hands—much like feeling for the popliteal pulse.

Findings

Similar to the considerations to make when examining a lump, during palpation of lymph nodes, standard features should be assessed:

Site

- Important diseases such as both acute and chronic infections and metastatic carcinoma will cause localized lymphadenopathy depending on the site of primary pathology.
- It is often helpful to draw a diagram detailing exactly where the enlarged node is. See Box 3.2 for causes of generalized lymphadenopathy.

Number

- How many nodes are enlarged?
- Make a diagram and detail the palpable nodes clearly and carefully.

Size

- Normal nodes are not palpable.
- Palpable nodes, therefore, are enlarged.
  - You should measure their length and width.

Consistency

- Malignant lymph nodes feel unusually firm or hard and irregular.
- Enlarged nodes secondary to infection may feel 'rubbery'.

Tenderness

- Painful, tender nodes usually imply infection.

Fixation

- Nodes that are fixed to surrounding tissue are highly suspicious of malignancy.
- Matted glands may occur in tuberculous lymphadenopathy.

Overlying skin

- Inflamed nodes may cause redness and swelling in the overlying skin.
- Spread of a metastatic carcinoma into the surrounding tissue may cause oedema and surface texture changes.

Box 3.2 Some causes of generalized lymphadenopathy

- Haematological malignancies (e.g. lymphoma, acute, and chronic lymphatic leukaemia)
- Infections:
  - Viral (e.g. HIV, infectious mononucleosis, CMV)
  - Bacterial (e.g. tuberculosis, syphilis, brucellosis)
- Infiltrative diseases (e.g. sarcoidosis, amyloidosis)
- Autoimmune diseases (e.g. systemic lupus erythematosus, rheumatoid arthritis)
- Drugs (e.g. phenytoin causes a 'pseudolymphoma').

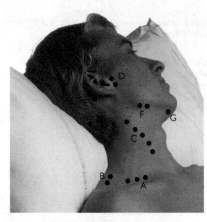

A = Supraclavicular
B = Posterior triangle
C = Jugular chain
D = Preauricular
E = Postauricular
F = Submandibular
G = Submental
H = Occipital

Fig. 3.1 Cervical and supraclavicular lymph nodes.

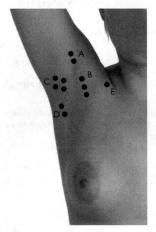

A = Lateral
B = Pectoral
C = Central
D = Subscapular
E = Infraclavicular

Fig. 3.2 Axillary lymph nodes.

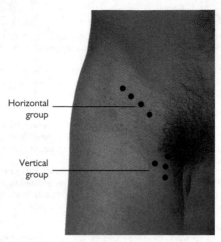

Fig. 3.3 Inguinal lymph nodes.

Hands and upper limbs

Examination of the hands is an important part of all examination routines and may provide a huge number of diagnostic clues. It is also something that the student may be asked to perform on a regular basis.

You will meet various 'hand signs' throughout this book.

Be sure to include assessment of:

- Both the dorsal surface and the palm.
- Skin colour.
- Discrete lesions.
- Muscles.
- Joints.
- Bony deformities.
- Nails.
- Remember to palpate and test movement and sensation.

After examining the hands, palpate both the radial and ulnar pulses.

Elbows

- Always examine the elbows to elicit any clues as to the cause of joint pathology.
- For example, there may be rheumatoid nodules, psoriatic plaques, xanthomata, or scars.

Recognizable syndromes

Some physical (especially facial) characteristics are so typical of certain congenital, endocrine, and other disorders that they immediately suggest the diagnosis.

Certain physical features of conditions can be appreciated on first inspection—enabling a 'spot diagnosis'. Most of these conditions have many other features which are not detailed here.

Down's syndrome (trisomy 21)

- *Facies:* oblique orbital fissures, epicanthic folds, hypertelorism (widely spaced eyes), conjunctivitis, lenticular opacities, small low-set ears, flat nasal bridge, mouth hanging open, protruding tongue (large, heavily fissured).
- *Hands:* single palmar crease (not pathognomonic), short broad hands, curved little finger, hyperflexible joints with generalized hypotonia.
- *Other:* mental deficiency, wide gap between 1st and 2nd toes, short stature, dementia of Alzheimer type, hypothyroidism.

Turner's syndrome (45 XO)

- *Facies:* micrognathia (small chin), epicanthic folds, low-set ears, fish-like mouth, hypertelorism, ptosis, strabismus.
- *Neck:* short, webbed neck, redundant skin folds at back of neck, low hairline.
- *Chest:* shield-like chest, widely spaced nipples.
- *Limbs:* short fourth metacarpal or metatarsal, hyperplastic nails, lymphoedema, increased carrying angle of the elbow.

Marfan's syndrome

Autosomal dominant condition caused by defects in fibrillin gene (ch15q).

- *Facies:* long, narrow face, high-arched palate, lens dislocation, heterochromia of iris, blue sclera, myopia.
- *Limbs:* tall stature, armspan > height, hyperextensibility of joints, recurrent dislocations.
- *Hands:* elongated fingers and toes (arachnodactyly).
- *Chest:* funnel or pigeon chest, kyphoscoliosis, aortic incompetence.
- *Other:* cystic disease of the lungs (spontaneous pneumothorax, bullae, apical fibrosis, aspergilloma and bronchiectasis), inguinal or femoral herniae.

Tuberous sclerosis

Also known as Bourneville's disease of the skin. Autosomal dominant condition localized to chromosomes 16 and 9.

- *Skin:* adenoma sebaceum (angiofibromata—papular, salmon-coloured eruption on centre of the face, especially at the nasolabial folds); shagreen patches (flesh-coloured, lumpy plaques found mostly on the lower back); ungal fibromata (firm, pink, periungual papules growing out from nail beds of fingers and toes); hypopigmented 'ash-leaf' macules (trunk and buttocks); café-au-lait macules and patches.

Neurofibromatosis type 1

Also known as von Recklinghausen's disease—autosomal dominant.

- *Skin:* neurofibromata (single, lobulated or pedunculated, soft, firm, mobile, lumps or nodules along the course of nerves), café-au-lait spots (especially in the axillae), axillary freckling.
- *Other:* kyphoscoliosis, nerve root involvement or compression, muscle wasting, sensory loss (Charcot's joints), plexiform neuroma, lung cysts.

Peutz–Jeghers syndrome

- *Skin:* sparse or profuse small brownish-black pigmented macules on lips, around mouth and on buccal mucosa, hands, and fingers.

Oculocutaneous albinism

- Marked hypomelanosis (pale skin), white hair or faintly yellow blonde.
- Nystagmus, photophobia, hypopigmented fundus, translucent (pink) iris.

Myotonic dystrophy*

- *Facies:* myopathic facies (drooping mouth and long, lean, sad, sleepy expression), frontal balding in men, ptosis, wasting of facial muscles (especially temporalis and masseter), cataracts.
- *Other:* wasting of sternomastoids, shoulder girdle, and quadriceps, areflexia, myotonia (percussion in tongue and thenar eminence, delay before releasing grip), cardiomyopathy, slurred speech, testicular atrophy, diabetes, intellect and personality deterioration in later stages.

Parkinson's disease*

- *Facies:* expressionless, unblinking face, drooling, titubation, blepharoclonus (tremor of eyelids when eyes gently closed).
- *Gait:* shuffling, festinant gait with reduced arm swing.
- *Tremor:* pill-rolling tremor, lead-pipe rigidity, cog-wheel rigidity, glabellar tap positive, small, tremulous, untidy hand writing (micrographia).

Osler–Weber–Rendu syndrome

Also known as hereditary haemorrhagic telangiectasia (HHT).

- *Facies:* telangiectasia (on face, around mouth, on lips, on tongue, buccal mucosa, nasal mucosa), telangiectasia may also be found on fingers. Associated with epistaxis, GI haemorrhage, iron-deficiency anaemia, haemoptysis.

Systemic sclerosis/CREST syndrome

- *Face/hands:* telangiectasia and pigmentation, pinched nose, perioral tethering, tight, shiny and adherent skin, vasculitis, atrophy of finger pulps, calcinosis (fingers), Raynaud's phenomenon.

* More detail in ➔ Chapter 8.

Vitamin and trace element deficiencies

Fat-soluble vitamins

Vitamin A (retinol)
- Found in dairy produce, eggs, fish oils, and liver.
- Deficiency causes night blindness, xerophthalmia, keratomalacia (corneal thickening), and follicular hyperkeratosis.

Vitamin D (cholecalciferol)
- Found in fish liver oils, dairy produce, and undergoes metabolism at the kidneys and the skin using UV light.
- Deficiency causes rickets (in children) and osteomalacia (in adults). Proximal muscle weakness may be evident.

Vitamin E (alpha-tocopherol)
- Widely distributed, green vegetables, and vegetable oils.
- Deficiency causes haemolytic anaemia (premature infants) and gross ataxia.

Vitamin K (K_1 = phylloquinine, K_2 = menaquinone)
- Widely distributed but particularly in green vegetables. Synthesized by intestinal bacteria.
- Deficiency causes coagulation defects seen as easy bruising and haemorrhage.

Water-soluble vitamins

Vitamin B_1 (thiamine)
- Found in cereals, peas, beans, yeast, and wholemeal flour. An essential factor in carbohydrate metabolism and transketolation reactions.
- Deficiency causes dry beri-beri (sensory and motor peripheral neuropathy), wet beri-beri (high output cardiac failure and oedema), and Wernicke–Korsakoff syndrome.

Vitamin B_2 (riboflavin)
- Found in wholemeal flour, meat, fish, and dairy produce. A coenzyme in reversible electron carriage in oxidation–reduction reactions.
- Deficiency gives angular stomatitis (fissuring and inflammation at the corners of the mouth), inflamed oral mucous membranes, seborrhoeic dermatitis, and peripheral neuropathy.

Vitamin B_3 (niacin)
- Found in fish, liver, nuts, and wholemeal flour.
- Deficiency causes pellagra: dermatitis, diarrhoea, and dementia.

Vitamin B_6 (pyridoxine)
- Widespread distribution, also synthesized from tryptophan.
- Deficiency causes peripheral neuropathy, convulsions, and sideroblastic anaemia. Deficiency may be provoked by a number of commonly used drugs (e.g. isoniazid, hydralazine, penicillamine) and is also seen in alcoholism and pregnancy.

Vitamin B₉ (folic acid)

- Deficiency can be caused by poor diet, malabsorption states, coeliac disease, Crohn's disease, gastrectomy, drugs (e.g. methotrexate, phenytoin), excessive utilization (e.g. leukaemia, malignancy, inflammatory disease).
- Consequences of deficiency include megaloblastic anaemia and glossitis.

Vitamin B₁₂ (cyanocobalamin)

- Causes of a deficiency are numerous and include partial or total gastrectomy, Crohn's disease, ileal resection, jejunal diverticulae, blind loop syndrome, and tapeworm.
- Deficiency causes megaloblastic anaemia, peripheral neuropathy, subacute combined degeneration of the spinal cord, depression, psychosis, and optic atrophy.

Vitamin C (ascorbic acid)

- Deficiency causes scurvy (perifollicular haemorrhage, bleeding swollen gums, spontaneous bruising, corkscrew hair, failure of wound healing), anaemia, and osteoporosis.

Trace elements

Copper

- Deficiency results in hypochromic and microcytic anaemia, neutropenia, impaired bone mineralization, Menkes' kinky hair syndrome (growth failure, mental deficiency, bone lesions, brittle hair, anaemia), sensory ataxia, muscle weakness, visual loss (optic neuropathy), peripheral neuropathy.
  - Usually caused by copper malabsorption.

Zinc

- Deficiency causes achondromatosis enterpathica (infants develop growth retardation, hair loss, severe diarrhoea, candida and bacterial infections), impaired wound healing, skin ulcers, alopecia, night blindness, confusion, apathy, and depression.

Magnesium

- Severe deficiency can cause cardiac arrhythmias, paraesthesia, and tetany.

Iodine

- Severe deficiency can cause cretinism (children), hypothyroidism, and goitre.

The elderly patient

For Nigel Hawthorne's on-screen King George III, examination by his doctor during an attack of porphyria was 'the very last resort' and viewed as an 'intolerable intrusion'. However, for older people, in whom the 'typical' presentations of illness may be subtle or unusual, a thorough physical examination is a cornerstone of assessment.

The value of a thorough physical examination can be underestimated by doctors, but be highly regarded as a therapeutic benefit by patients. This general overview complements the system-based chapters that follow, but the key message is repeated throughout—to reinforce the value of a comprehensive, holistic, and unrushed examination.

General points

Use your eyes
- A key question in your mind should be 'is the patient unwell?'
- Learn not to overlook key indices such as hypothermia and delirium which point to an acutely unwell patient.

Seek additional diagnoses
- Multiple illnesses are a typical feature of old age—seemingly incidental findings (to the presenting condition) are common, so look out for such things as:
  - Skin lesions (malignant?)
  - New/isolated patches of 'psoriasis' (Bowen's disease?)
  - Asymptomatic peripheral arterial disease.

Talk to your patient
- During the examination as well as during the history.
- As indicated, it is often of huge therapeutic benefit, of reassurance, engendering trust, and potentially gaining additional history— especially if an incidental lesion is discovered.

Key points

Observations
- Nurses spend time recording them—so do your colleagues the courtesy of recording them in the notes, *and act on them.*
- Many patients may run low blood pressures, often as a consequence of medications—a small drop from this point is easily overlooked, but may be the only sign of a myocardial infarction.
- Recognize the limits of temperature/fever—seriously unwell older people may actually be hypothermic.
- Recognize the limits of early warning scores for older people, especially with chronic diseases as you may be falsely reassured.

Hydration
- May be difficult to assess—reduction in skin turgor through changes in elasticity with age, dry mucous membranes (e.g. through mouth breathing), or sunken eyes (muscle wasting, weight loss) are useful in younger patients, but less reliable in elders.
  - ▶ A useful alternative is axillary palpation—are they sweating?

Skin and nail health
- Asteatosis and varicose eczema are common, but easily overlooked.
- Look out for typical lesions in atypical places—squamous cell carcinomas are notorious in this respect.
- Learn to look at footwear/toenails—is there onychogryphosis?

Nutrition
- Signs of weight loss are often obvious—ill-fitting clothes and dentures are good examples.

Joints
- Remember to look and examine—is the patient's mobility worse, or the reason for falling acute (pseudo) gout?

MMSE/AMTS
- Should be mandatory for the majority of patients.

Gait (where possible)
- Akin to mental state examination, should be undertaken whenever possible. See ⮞ Chapter 10 for the 'get up and go' test.

Geriatric giants
So described by Bernard Isaacs, one of the key figures of contemporary geriatric medicine. Isaacs described five 'giants':
▶ These are not 'diagnoses', so avoid reaching them—but extremely common presentations of illness in older people, for which an underlying cause (or causes!) should be sought.
- Immobility.
- Instability.
- Incontinence.
- Intellectual impairment.
- Iatrogenic illness.

Information gathering
Faced with an acutely unwell, delirious patient, no old notes or GP letter and 'little to go on', it can be tempting to fall back on Isaacs' giants as a diagnosis. Make that extra effort to enquire of others for information which will reveal vital clues:
- Family and carers (e.g. care home staff): a real opportunity to update family, reassure or open up a conversation about other issues.
- IT: virtually all hospitals allow access to e-systems that record clinic letters, discharge notes, and results.
- GP surgeries: both for the Summary Care Record/current prescription and a discussion with one of the GPs, who is likely to know the patient better than you.
- Community services: you will often find that the rest of the multi-disciplinary team are ahead of you in liaising and gathering important information from homecare, district nurses, and intermediate care.

Symptoms in endocrinology

As hormones have an impact on every body system, it is therefore necessary to cover all areas of general health in history taking.

This section outlines some of the more important presenting symptoms in endocrine disease which should not be missed (if a high index of clinical suspicion is held regarding endocrine dysfunction), but it is by no means exhaustive.

Appetite and weight changes

Many people do not weigh themselves but may have noticed the consequences of weight change such as clothes becoming looser or tighter.

Lethargy

Lethargy or fatigue is a difficult symptom to pin down. Ask the patient how the tiredness impacts on their daily life. What are they able to do before needing to rest—and has this changed? Fatigue may be a feature of undiagnosed endocrine disease such as:

- Diabetes mellitus.
- Cushing's syndrome.
- Hypoadrenalism.
- Hypothyroidism.
- Hypercalcaemia.

▶ Consider depression and chronic disease of any other kind (anaemia, chronic liver and renal problems, chronic infection, and malignancy).

Bowel habit

Constipation is a common feature of hypercalcaemia and hypothyroidism. Hyperthyroidism and Addison's disease may give diarrhoea.

Urinary frequency and polyuria

Endocrine causes might include:

- Diabetes mellitus.
- Diabetes insipidus.
- Hyperglycaemia caused by Cushing's syndrome.
- Polyuria may also be seen in the presence of hypercalcaemia.

Thirst and polydipsia

Consider diabetes mellitus, diabetes insipidus, and hypercalcaemia.

Sweating

↑ perspiration may be seen during episodes of hypoglycaemia as well as in hyperthyroidism and acromegaly, and is associated with the other adrenergic symptoms of a phaeochromocytoma.

Pigmentation

Localized loss of pigmentation may be due to vitiligo—an autoimmune disorder associated with other endocrine immune diseases such as hypo- or hyperthyroidism, Addison's disease, and Hashimoto's thyroiditis.

- ↑ *pigmentation:* Addison's disease, Cushing's syndrome.
- ↓ *pigmentation:* generalized loss of pigmentation in hypopituitarism.

Hair distribution

Hair loss

Decreased adrenal androgen production and loss of axillary and pubic hair in both sexes can be caused by:

- Hypogonadism.
- Adrenal insufficiency.

Hair gain

Hirsutism or excessive hair growth in a female may be due to endocrine dysfunction. Consider:

- Polycystic ovarian syndrome.
- Cushing's syndrome.
- Congenital adrenal hyperplasia.
- Acromegaly.
- Virilizing tumours.

Skin and soft tissue changes

Endocrine disorders cause many soft tissue changes including:

- *Hypothyroidism:* dry, coarse, pale skin with xanthelasma formation and, classically, loss of the outer 1/3 of the eyebrows.
- *Hyperthyroidism:* thyroid acropachy is seen only in hyperthyroidism due to Graves' disease. Features include finger clubbing and new bone formation at the fingers. Also pretibial myxoedema—reddened oedematous lesions on the shins (often the lateral aspects).
- *Hypoparathyroidism:* generally dry, scaly skin.
- *Diabetes mellitus:* xanthelasma, ulceration, repeated skin infections, necrobiosis lipoidica diabeticorum—shiny, yellowed lesions on the shins.
- *Acromegaly:* soft tissue overgrowth with skin tags at the axillae and anus, 'doughy' hands and fingers, acanthosis nigricans—velvety black skin changes at the axilla. (Acanthosis nigricans can also be seen in Cushing's syndrome, polycystic ovarian syndrome, and insulin resistance.)

Headache and visual disturbance

Visual field defects, cranial nerve palsies, and headache may be caused by space-occupying lesions within the skull. Pituitary tumours classically cause a bitemporal hemianopia by impinging on the optic chiasm.

Blurred vision is rather non-specific, but consider osmotic changes in the lens due to hyperglycaemia.

Alteration in growth

Hypopituitarism, hypothyroidism, growth hormone deficiency, and steroid excess may present with short stature. Tall stature may be caused by growth hormone excess or gonadotrophin deficiency.

Growth hormone excess in adults (acromegaly) causes soft tissue overgrowth. Patients may notice an increase in shoe size, glove size, or facial appearance (do they have any old photographs for comparison?).

Changes in sexual function
Women
Altered menstrual pattern in a female may be an early symptom suggestive of pituitary dysfunction.

Men
In men, hypogonadism may result in loss of libido and an inability to attain or sustain an erection.
► Remember to look for non-endocrine causes of sexual dysfunction such as alcoholism, spinal cord disease, or psychological illness.

Flushing
Flushing may be a symptom of carcinoid or the menopause.
Ask about the nature of the flushing, any aggravating or relieving factors, and, importantly, any other symptoms at the time such as palpitations, diarrhoea, dizziness. Remember to take a full menstrual history.

The rest of the history

A full history should be taken (see Box 3.3 for the history in patients with diabetes). In a patient with endocrine symptoms, you should pay special attention to the following:

Drug history
As ever, a detailed medication history should be sought. Remember to ask especially about:
- Over-the-counter (OTC) medicines.
- Hormonal treatments—including the oral contraceptive pill, local, and systemic steroids.
- Amiodarone.
- Lithium.
- Herbal or other remedies.

Past medical history
- Any previous thyroid or parathyroid surgery.
- Any previous [131]I (radio-iodine) treatment or antithyroid drugs.
- Gestational diabetes.
- Hypertension.
- Any previous pituitary or adrenal surgery.

Family history
Ask especially about:
- Type II diabetes (Box 3.3).
- Related autoimmune disorders (pernicious anaemia, coeliac disease, vitiligo, Addison's disease, thyroid disease, type I diabetes).
  - Many patients will only have heard of these if they have a family member who suffers from them.
- Congential adrenal hyperplasia (CAH).
- Tumours of the MEN syndromes (Box 3.4).

Box 3.3 The diabetic history

As with other diseases, you should establish when the diagnosis was made (and how) and the course and treatment of the disease. There are additional questions relating to disease monitoring and diabetic complications that you should ask patients with diabetes:

- When was it first diagnosed?
- How was it first diagnosed?
- How was it first managed?
- How is it managed now?
- If on insulin—when was that first started?
- Are they compliant with a diabetic diet?
- Are they compliant with their diabetic medication?
- How often do they check their blood sugar?
- What readings do they normally get (if possible, ask to see their monitoring booklet)?
- What is their latest Hb_A1_c (many will know this)?
- Have they ever been admitted to hospital with diabetic ketoacidosis (DKA)?
- Do they go to a podiatrist or chiropodist?
- Have they experienced any problems with their feet? Do they use any moisturizers or cream on their feet?
- Do they attend a retinal screening program?
- Have they needed to be referred to an ophthalmologist?

If the patient is newly diagnosed with diabetes, ask about a history of weight loss (may differentiate type I and type II diabetes).

Box 3.4 The MEN syndromes

'Multiple endocrine neoplasias' which display autosomal dominant inheritance.

MEN 1

The 3 Ps:

- Parathyroid hyperplasia (100%)
- Pancreatic endocrine tumours (40–70%)
- Pituitary adenomas (30–50%).

MEN 2

- Medullary cell thyroid carcinoma (100%)
- Phaeochromocytoma (50%) and...
  - MEN 2a: parathyroid hyperplasia (80%)
  - MEN 2b: mucosal and bowel neuromas, marfanoid habitus.

General endocrine examination

It is not possible to perform an examination of the endocrine system in the same way that you may examine other organ systems. Usually, an endocrine examination is focused—looking for signs to confirm or refute differential diagnoses that you have developed.

See Box 3.5 for signs of tetany.

You may, however, perform a quick 'screening' general examination of a patient's endocrine status.

Hands/arms

Look at size, subcutaneous tissue, length of the metacarpals, nails, palmar erythema, sweating, and tremor. Note also skin thickness (thin skin in Cushing's, thick skin in acromegaly) and look for signs of easy bruising.

Pulse and blood pressure—lying and standing. Test for proximal muscle weakness.

Axillae

Note any skin tags, loss of hair, abnormal pigmentation, or acanthosis nigricans.

Face and mouth

Look for hirsutism, acne, plethora, or skin greasiness. Look at the soft tissues of the face for prominent glabellas (above the eyes) and enlargement of the chin (macrognathism). In the mouth, look at the spacing of the teeth and if any have fallen out. Note any buccal pigmentation and tongue enlargement (macroglossia). Normally, the upper teeth close in front of the lower set—reversal of this is termed 'prognathism'.

Neck

Note any swellings or lymphadenopathy. Examine the thyroid. Palpate the supraclavicular regions and note excessive soft tissue.

Chest

Inspect for any hair excess or loss, breast size in females and gynaecomastia in males. Note the nipple colour, pigmentation, or galactorrhoea.

Abdomen

Inspect for central adiposity/obesity, purple striae, hirsutism. Palpate for organomegaly. Look at the external genitalia to exclude any testicular atrophy in males or virilization (e.g. clitoromegaly) in women.

Legs

Test for proximal muscle weakness and make note of any diabetes-related changes.

Height and weight

Calculate the patient's BMI.

Box 3.5 Signs of tetany

Trousseau's sign

Inflate a blood pressure cuff just above the systolic pressure for 3 minutes. When hypocalcaemia has caused muscular irritability, the hand will develop flexor spasm.

Chvostek's sign

Gently tap over the facial nerve (in front of the tragus of the ear). The sign is positive if there is contraction of the lip and facial muscles on the same side of the face.

Examining the thyroid

The patient should be sitting upright on a chair or the edge of a bed.

Inspection

Look at the thyroid region. If the gland is quite enlarged (goitre), you may notice it protruding as a swelling just below the thyroid cartilage. The normal thyroid gland is usually neither visible nor palpable.

Thyroid gland

The gland lies ~2–3cm below the thyroid cartilage and has 2 equal lobes connected by a narrow isthmus.

If a localized or generalized swelling is visible, ask the patient to take a mouthful of water then swallow—watch the neck swelling carefully. Also ask the patient to protrude their tongue and watch the neck swelling.

- The thyroid is attached to the thyroid cartilage of the larynx and will move up with swallowing.
- Other neck masses such as an enlarged lymph node will hardly move.
- Thyroglossal cysts will not move with swallowing but will move upwards with protrusion of the tongue.

The rest of the neck

- Carefully inspect the neck for any obvious scars (thyroidectomy scars are often hidden below a necklace and are easily missed).
- Look for the JVP and make note of dilated veins which may indicate retrosternal extension of a goitre.
- Redness or erythema may indicate suppurative thyroiditis.

Palpation

Thyroid gland

Always begin palpation from behind. Stand behind the patient and place a hand either side of their neck. The patient's neck should be slightly flexed to relax the sternomastoids. ❶ Explain what you are doing.

- Ask if there is any tenderness.
- Place the middle 3 fingers of either hand along the midline of the neck, just below the chin.
- Gently 'walk' your fingers down until you reach the thyroid gland.
  - The central isthmus is almost never palpable
- If the gland is enlarged, determine if it is symmetrical.
- Are there any discrete nodules?
- Assess the size, shape, and mobility of any swelling.
- Repeat the examination whilst the patient swallows.
  - Ask them to hold a small amount of water in their mouth—then ask them to swallow once your hands are in position.
- Consider the consistency of any palpable thyroid tissue:
  - Soft: normal
  - Firm: simple goitre
  - Rubbery hard: Hashimoto's thyroiditis
  - Stony hard: cancer, cystic calcification, fibrosis, Riedel's thyroiditis.
- Feel for a palpable thrill which may be present in metabolically active thyrotoxicosis.

The rest of the neck

Palpate cervical lymph nodes, carotid arteries (to check for patency—can be compressed by a large thyroid) and the trachea for deviation.

Percussion

- Percuss downwards from the sternal notch.
- In retrosternal enlargement the percussion note over the manubrosternum is dull as opposed to the normal resonance.

Auscultation

Apply the diaphragm of the stethoscope over each lobe of the thyroid gland and auscultate for a bruit.

- A soft bruit is indicative of increased blood flow which is characteristic of the hyperthyroid goitre seen in Graves' disease.
  - You may need to occlude venous return within the IJV to rule out a venous hum
  - Listen over the aortic area to ensure that the thyroid bruit is not, in fact, an outflow obstruction murmur conducted to the root of the neck.

Skills station 3.1

Instruction

Clinically assess this patient's thyroid status.

Model technique

- Clean your hands.
- Introduce yourself.
- Explain the purpose of examination, obtain informed consent.
- Ask for any painful areas you should avoid.
- Observe the patient's composure (relaxed/agitated/fidgety?).
- Measure the heart rate and note if the patient is in atrial fibrillation.
- Inspect the hands—erythema, warmth, thyroid acropachy (phalangeal bone overgrowth similar to pulmonary osteopathy).
- Feel the palms—sweaty/dry?
- Look for peripheral tremor—ask the patient to stretch out their arms with fingers out straight and palms down. Resting a piece of paper on the back of the hand can make a tremor more obvious.
- Inspect the face.
  - Exophthalmos, proptosis.
  - Hypothyroid features.
- Examine the eyes.
- Examine the thyroid and neck.
- Test tendon reflexes at the biceps and ankle.
- Test for proximal myopathy by asking the patient to stand from a sitting position.
- Look for pretibial myxoedema.
- Thank the patient and help them re-dress as necessary.

Examining the patient with diabetes

As diabetes has an impact on every body system, you can make the examination of a diabetic patient complex or simple depending on the circumstance.

In general, you should be alert to: cardiovascular disease, renal disease, retinal disease, peripheral neuropathy—especially sensory, health of insulin injection sites, the diabetic foot, secondary causes of diabetes (e.g. acromegaly, Cushing's syndrome, haemochromatosis), and associated hyperlipidaemia.

Framework for a thorough diabetic examination

General inspection
- Hydration.
- Weight.
- Facies associated with a known endocrine disease.
- Pigmentation (hyperpigmentation or patchy loss).

Legs
- Muscle wasting.
- Hair loss.
- Skin atrophy.
- Skin pigmentation.
- Leg ulceration (especially around pressure points and toes).
- Skin infections.

Injection sites
- Inspect and palpate for fat atrophy, fat hypertrophy, or local infection.

Associated skin lesions
- Necrobiosis lipoidica diabeticorum—look on the shins, arms, and back.
  - Sharply demarcated oval plaques with a shiny surface, yellow waxy atrophic centres, brownish-red margins, surrounding telangiectasia.
- Also look for granuloma annulare.

Hyperlipidaemia
- Eruptive xanthoma.
- Tendon xanthoma.
- Xanthelasma.

Neurological examination
- Visual acuity.
- Fundoscopy.
- Peripheral sensory neuropathy—evidence of injury, ulceration, and Charcot's joint formation.
- Test muscle strength.
- Examine feet.

Cardiovascular examination
- Ideally a full cardiovascular examination including lying and standing blood pressure measurements.

The diabetic foot

The combination of peripheral vascular disease and peripheral neuropathy can lead to repeated minor trauma to the feet leading to ulceration and infection which are very slow to heal.

Using a 10g monofilament
A small, thin plastic filament, designed such that it bends under approximately 10g of pressure.
- Apply the filament to the patient's skin at the spots shown in Fig. 3.4a.
- Press firmly so that the filament bends (Fig. 3.4b).
- Hold the filament against the skin for ~1.5 seconds and ask the patient if they can feel it. The filament should not slide, stroke, or scratch.
- ❗ Do not press on ulcers, callouses, scars, or necrotic tissue.
  - The patient's feet are 'at risk' if they cannot feel the monofilament at any of the sites.

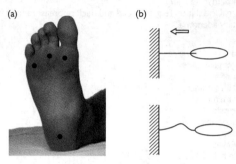

Fig. 3.4 (a) Sites to test with a 10g monofilament in the diabetic patient. (b) Apply the monofilament to the skin with enough force to make it bend.

Skills station 3.2

Instruction
Clinically assess the foot of this patient with diabetes.

Model technique
- Clean your hands.
- Introduce yourself.
- Explain the purpose of examination, obtain informed consent.
- Inspect, noting colour, ulceration, dryness, callous formation, evidence of infection.
- Evidence of injury—shoes rubbing?
- Are there any Charcot's joints?
  - Grossly abnormal and dysfunctional joints due to repeated minor trauma and poor healing due to a loss of pain sensation.
- 10g monofilament test.
- Test light-touch sensation, pain sensation, vibration sense, and proprioception.
- Palpate the peripheral pulses (dorsalis pedis and posterior tibial).
- Note the temperature of the skin on the dorsum and sole.
- Record capillary filling time.
- Thank the patient and help them re-dress as necessary.

Important presentations

Hypothyroidism

Causes

- Dietary iodine deficiency.
- Autoimmune thyroiditis (Hashimoto's thyroiditis).
- Lymphocytic thyroiditis (10% of post-partum women).
- Drugs (amiodarone, interferon alpha, thalidomide, dopamine, lithium).
- Radioactive iodine treatment.
- Surgical thyroid injury.
- External irradiation (e.g. for head and neck or breast cancer).
- Pituitary adenoma.

Symptoms

- Tiredness.
- Weight gain.
- Anorexia.
- Cold intolerance.
- Poor memory.
- Depression.
- Reduced libido.
- Goitre.
- Puffy eyes.
- Brittle hair.
- Dry skin.
- Arthralgia.
- Myalgia.
- Muscle weakness.
- Constipation.
- Menorrhagia.

Signs

- *General:* croaking voice, mental and physical sluggishness, pseudodementia, 'myxoedema madness'.
- *Inspection:* coarse cool dry skin (look for yellowish tint of carotenaemia 'peaches and cream' complexion), palmar crease pallor, peripheral cyanosis, puffy lower eyelids, loss of outer 1/3 of eyebrows, thinning of scalp hair, tongue swelling, xanthelasma.
- *Cardiovascular and chest:* mild hypertension, pericarditis, pleural effusion, low cardiac output, cardiac failure, bradycardia, small volume pulse.
- *Neurological:* carpal tunnel syndrome, peripheral neuropathy, cerebellar syndrome, proximal muscle weakness, myotonia, muscular hypertrophy, delayed ankle jerks, bilateral neural deafness (seen in congenital hypothyroidism).

Hyperthyroidism

Causes
- Graves' disease.
- Chronic thyroiditis (Hashimoto thyroiditis).
- Subacute thyroiditis (de Quervain thyroiditis).
- Postpartum thyroiditis.
- Drugs (iodine-induced, amiodarone).
- Bacterial thyroiditis.
- Postviral thyroiditis.
- Idiopathic.
- Toxic multinodular goitre.
- Malignancy (toxic adenoma, TSH-producing pituitary tumours).

Symptoms
- Weight loss.
- Increased appetite.
- Irritability.
- Restlessness.
- Muscle weakness.
- Tremor.
- Breathlessness.
- Palpitations.
- Sweating.
- Heat intolerance.
- Itching.
- Thirst.
- Vomiting.
- Diarrhoea.
- Eye complaints (Graves' ophthalmopathy).
- Oligomenorrhoea.
- Loss of libido.
- Gynaecomastia.

Signs:
- *General:* irritability, weight loss.
- *Inspection:* onycholysis, palmar erythema, tremor, sweaty palms, thyroid acropachy, hyperkinesis, gynaecomastia, pretibial myxoedema, Graves' ophthalmopathy.
- *Cardiovascular and chest:* resting tachycardia, high cardiac output, systolic flow murmurs.
- *Neurological:* proximal myopathy, muscle wasting, hyper-reflexia in legs.

Glucocorticoid excess (Cushing's syndrome)

- *Causes include:* high ACTH production from a pituitary adenoma and ectopic ACTH (e.g. small cell lung cancer). Primary hypercortisolaemia caused by adrenal hyperplasia, adrenal tumour (adenoma or carcinoma), exogenous steroids; ectopic CRF production (very rare), depression, alcohol-induced.
- *Symptoms:* weight gain (central/upper body), change in appearance, menstrual disturbance, thin skin with easy bruising, acne, excessive hair growth, muscle weakness, decreased libido, depression, insomnia.
- *Signs:* supraclavicular fat pads, 'moon face', thoracocervical fat pads ('buffalo hump'), centripetal obesity, hirsutism, thinning of skin, easy bruising, purple striae, poor wound healing, skin infections, proximal muscle weakness (shoulders and hips), ankle oedema, hypertension, fractures due to osteoporosis, hyperpigmentation (if raised ACTH), glycosuria.

Hypoadrenalism (Addison's disease)

- *Causes include:* autoimmune adrenalitis (>80% in UK), tuberculosis, metastatic malignancy, amyloidosis, haemorrhage, infarction, bilateral adrenalectomy, HIV.
- *Symptoms:* anorexia, weight loss, tiredness, nausea, vomiting, diarrhoea, constipation, abdominal pain, confusion, erectile dysfunction, amenorrhoea, dizziness, syncope, myalgia, arthralgia.
- *Signs:* skin pigmentation (especially on sun-exposed areas, mucosal surfaces, axillae, palmar creases, and in recent scars), cachexia, loss of body hair, postural hypotension, low-grade fever, dehydration.

Growth hormone excess (acromegaly)

- *Causes:* pituitary tumour (>95%), hyperplasia due to GHRH excess (very rare), tumours in hypothalamus, adrenal, or pancreas.
- *Symptoms:* headache, diplopia, change in appearance, enlarged extremities, deepening of voice, sweating, tiredness, weight gain, erectile dysfunction, dysmenorrhoea, galactorrhoea, snoring, arthralgia, weakness, numbness, paraesthesia, polyuria, polydipsia.
- *Signs:* prominent supraorbital ridges, large nose and lips, protrusion of lower jaw (prognathism), interdental separation, macroglossia, 'spade-like' hands, 'doughy' soft tissues, thick oily skin, carpal tunnel syndrome, hirsutism, bitemporal hemianopia (if pituitary tumour impinging on optic chiasm), cranial nerve palsies (particularly III, IV, and VI), hypertension.

Prolactinoma

A pituitary tumour (the most common hormone-secreting tumour).

- *Symptoms:* depend on age, sex, and degree of prolactinaemia. In females: oligomenorrhagia, vaginal dryness, dyspareunia, galactorrhoea. In males: loss of libido, erectile dysfunction, infertility, galactorrhoea. If before puberty, may have female body habitus and small testicles.
- *Signs:* visual field defects (bitemporal hemianopia?), cranial nerve palsies (III, IV, and VI), galactorrhoea. In males: small testicles and female pattern of hair growth.

Hypercalcaemia

- *Causes:* common—hyperparathyroidism, malignancy (PTHrP production or metastases in bone). Less common—vitamin D intoxication, granulomatous disease, familial hypocalciuric hypercalaemia. Rare—drugs (e.g. bendrofluazide), hyperthyroidism, Addison's disease.
- *Symptoms:* depend largely on the underlying cause. Mild hypercalcaemia is asymptomatic. Higher levels may cause nausea, vomiting, drowsiness, confusion, abdominal pain, constipation, depression, muscle weakness, myalgia, polyuria, headache, and coma.
- *Signs:* often there are signs of the underlying cause. There are no specific signs of hypercalcaemia.

Hypocalcaemia

- *Causes:* hypoalbuminaemia, hypomagnesaemia, hyperphosphataemia, surgery to the thyroid or parathyroid glands, PTH deficiency or resistance, and vitamin D deficiency.
- *Symptoms:* depression, paraesthesia around the mouth, muscle spasms.
- *Signs:* carpopedal spasm (flexion at the wrist and the fingers) when blood supply to the hand is reduced by inflating a sphygmomanometer cuff on the arm (Trousseau's sign). Nervous excitability—tapping a nerve causes the supplied muscles to twitch (Chvostek's sign—tapping facial nerve at the parotid gland about 2cm anterior to the tragus of the ear causes the facial muscles to contract).

Polycystic ovarian syndrome (PCOS)

Abnormal metabolism of androgens and oestrogen with abnormal control of androgen production.

- *Symptoms:* oligomenorrhoea with anovulation and erratic periods, infertility. Some patients present complaining of hirsutism.
- *Signs:* obesity (50%), male-pattern hair growth, male-pattern baldness, increased muscle mass, deep voice, clitoromegaly, acanthosis nigricans.

Practical procedures

Using this chapter

- This chapter describes those practical procedures that the junior doctor or senior nurse may be expected to perform.
- Obviously, some of these are more complicated than others—and should only be performed once you have been trained specifically in the correct technique by a more senior colleague.

Rules are made to be broken

- Very many procedures and practical skills do not have a 'correct' method but have an 'accepted' method.
- These methods should, therefore, be abided by but deviation from the routine by a competent practitioner, when circumstances demand, is acceptable.

Infiltrating anaesthetic agents

A large number of procedures involve the infiltration of local anaesthetic agents. It is important that you deliver these safely—injection of a large amount of anaesthetic into a vein could lead to potentially fatal cardiac arrhythmias. It is also important, of course, to ensure that you do not damage any vessels.

Advance and pull back

- Whenever you inject anything, you should advance the needle and attempt to pull back the plunger at each step—if you do not aspirate blood, you may *then* go ahead and infiltrate the anaesthetic.

Making a surface bleb

- Take the syringe of anaesthetic (e.g. 1% lidocaine = 10mg/ml) and a small needle.
- Pinch a portion of skin, insert the needle horizontally into the surface.
- Withdraw, as above, and inject a small amount of the anaesthetic—you should see a wheal of fluid rise.
- The area of skin will now be sufficiently anaesthetized to allow you to infiltrate deeper.

Other notes on local anaesthetics

- The maximum does of lidocaine is 3mg/kg in an adult.
  - This can be increased to 7mg/kg if mixed with adrenaline (although never to be used in this way at end-arteries).
- Lidocaine is a weak base and only works in its non-ionized form. It is, therefore, relatively ineffectual in infected (acidic) tissue.
- Lidocaine and other local anaesthetics sting on initial infiltration so warn the patient.

Hand hygiene

When?
The WHO World Alliance for Patient Safety, in 2006, identified 'five moments' for hand hygiene. These are:
- Before patient contact.
- Before an aseptic task.
- After body fluid exposure risk.
- After patient contact.
- After contact with a patient's surroundings.

Soap or alcohol gel?
Repeated washing with soap and water can cause skin dryness and can be time consuming. For these reasons, alcohol gel has become commonplace in clinical settings. There are no hard and fast rules but:
- Alcohol gel should not substitute soap and water if your hands are visibly soiled or if you are undertaking an aseptic procedure.
- Remember that alcohol gel is not effective against *Clostridium difficile*.

Soap and water technique
- Adhere to the 'bare below elbow' rule.
- Wet hands with water.
- Apply soap (from a dispenser) to cover all hand surfaces.
- Ensure all seven parts of the hands are thoroughly cleaned:
  - Rub hands palm-to-palm
  - Rub back of each hand with the palm of the other, fingers interlaced
  - Rub hands palm-to-palm with fingers interlaced
  - Lock hands together and rub backs of fingers against opposite palm
  - Rub thumbs in rotational movement with opposite hand
  - Rub tips of fingers into opposite palms
  - Rub each wrist with opposite hand.
- Hold hands under running water, rub vigorously to remove all suds.
- Turn off taps using elbows.
- Dry thoroughly with paper towel.
- Dispose of paper towels in appropriate clinical bin (using foot pedal).
- DO NOT TOUCH any other objects until task is undertaken and completed.

Alcohol gel technique
Essentially the same technique as above but no need to rinse or dry with a paper towel.
- Squirt small amount of gel onto centre of palm.
- Ensure all seven parts of the hands are thoroughly cleaned as above.
- Allow 20–30 seconds for hands to dry, holding hands up.
- Following disinfection, DO NOT TOUCH any other objects prior to commencing procedure.

Consent

See the latest guidance at ➫ http://www.gmc-uk.org

Introduction

Consent is permission granted by a person allowing you to subject them to something; anything from physical examination to surgical procedures. Performing an act on a competent adult without their consent constitutes a criminal offence. (See also Boxes 4.1 and 4.2.)

Capacity

The patient must be able to understand what a procedure involves, the possible consequences of a decision or of failure to make a decision. All adults are assumed to have capacity unless demonstrated otherwise.

Assessing capacity

The patient must be able to:
- Understand the information including any consequences.
- Retain the information.
- Weigh the information as part of decision making.
- Communicate their decision.

A patient lacking capacity

- Your reasons for believing a patient lacks capacity to make a certain decision should be clearly documented.
  - A patient may become temporarily incapacitated by, for example, acute confusion. Treatment may only be carried out in these circumstances if it cannot reasonably be delayed until incapacity is resolved. If this is the case, treatment must be decided according to the best interests of the patient.

Voluntary consent

- Consent is only valid if given voluntarily, without pressure from relatives, friends, or medical professionals.

Information

Patients must be provided with sufficient information to enable them to make an informed decision. Information must include:
- What the procedure entails and the rationale for doing it.
- Any alternatives available.
- Significant risks.
  - This includes any 'significant risk which would affect the judgement of a reasonable patient', not just those risks deemed significant by a responsible body of medical opinion (the Bolam test). Failure to disclose such risks may render you guilty of negligence.
- Additional procedures that may be necessary under the same anaesthetic should be discussed during initial consent.
- If patients refuse information about a procedure, this should be clearly documented and the patient provided with the opportunity to discuss later.

Consent forms
- Written consent is evidence that consent has been sought but does not confirm its validity.
- If consent is not voluntary, information is lacking, or the patient lacks capacity, then consent is not valid regardless of the presence of a consent form.
  - Certain procedures (included in the Mental Health Act and Human Fertilisation and Embryology Act) require written consent.
- ▶ Consent that is oral or non-verbal may also be valid.

Who should seek consent?
- Ideally, the professional providing the treatment or investigation in question, though this is not always possible.
- The professional seeking consent should at least have sufficient knowledge to understand and explain the procedure, its indication, and any risks involved.
  - If you are asked to seek consent for a procedure but lack this knowledge, it is your responsibility to seek advice from colleagues; failure to do so may result in invalid consent.

Refusal to consent
- If an adult with capacity refuses to give consent for a procedure, this must be respected (except in specific circumstances outlined in the Mental Health Act), even if refusal will lead to death of the patient or their unborn child.
- In these circumstances, rigorous examination of a patient's competence is necessary.
  - The same is true if a patient withdraws consent at any time, if they still have capacity.

Advanced refusal
- Advance refusal is valid if made at a time when a patient is competent and appropriately informed.
- Applicable when patient lacks capacity.
- Failure to respect the refusal may result in legal action.
- If doubt exists as to validity, the courts must be consulted.

Adults lacking capacity
- May be temporary, permanent, or fluctuating.
- ▶ No-one may give consent on behalf of an incompetent adult, unless a valid Lasting Power of Attorney exists.
- ▶ Patients must be treated in their best interests (not just medical interests) taking into account psychological, religious/spiritual, and financial well-being.
- Those close to the patient should be involved unless the patient has previously made clear that they should not be; independent patient advocacy services exist for consultation when the patient does not have anyone close.
- Where there is doubt as to best interests or capacity, the High Court may give a ruling.

Lasting powers of attorney (Mental Capacity Act 2005)

- A document created by someone (the 'donor') to confer authority to give consent for investigation or treatment (as well as other issues) to a named individual(s) ('donees').
- Must be registered.
- Only valid when the patient lacks capacity.
- Must specifically authorize the donee to make decisions regarding welfare or medical treatment.
  - ▶ Unless specifically stated, do not extend to decisions about life-sustaining treatment.

Patients under 18 years of age

16–17 years
- If competent, may consent to or refuse an intervention.
- If incompetent, an individual with parental responsibility may provide consent.

Under 16: Gillick competence
- A child under 16 may consent to treatment if they are able to fully understand what is involved in an intervention.
  - This may apply to some interventions and not others.
- If a child is Gillick competent, parental consent is not required, though it is good practice to encourage a child to inform their parents unless this is not in their best interests.

Overriding decisions: under 18 years
- Refusal may be overridden by an individual with parental responsibility or the courts.
- Should consider the person's welfare as a whole. May involve sharing information that the child does not wish divulged; necessary if refusal puts the child at serious risk.
- ▶ In dire emergency, where a person with parental responsibility is unreachable or refuses consent for life-saving treatment that appears to be in the best interests of the child, it is acceptable to preserve life.

Box 4.1 Pre-procedure ABCDE

Questions to ask yourself before any procedure:
- A = Allergies
- B = Bloods
- C = Consent
- D = Drug history
- E = Emergency cover in case of complication or failure of the procedure.

Box 4.2 WHO checklist

- The WHO pre-procedure checklist is a series of questions to ask of the patient and the person performing the procedure
- This is usually reserved for complex interventional procedures and surgery
  - Check your local guidance
- Questions cover introductions, patient details, allergies, details of the procedure and any other pre-procedure checks
  - You should familiarize yourself with the questions and perform these checks yourself before performing any procedure (even if not on a formal WHO checklist form)
- For more information, go to ℘ http://www.who.int

Aseptic technique

▶ You should always consider the sterility of the items to be touched before you begin each procedure. If some or all items need to remain sterile, an aseptic technique should be used.

Aseptic non-touch technique

The highest level of asepsis, designed to minimize or completely remove the chance of contamination, is known as 'aseptic non-touch technique' (ANTT) (Boxes 4.3 and 4.4).

Before
- Wash hands with soap and water or alcohol gel.
- Put on disposable apron and any other protective items.
- Clean trolley/tray with wipes and dry with a paper towel.
- Gather equipment and put on the lower shelf of the trolley.
- Take trolley/tray to the patient.

During
- Wash hands with alcohol gel.
- Remove sterile pack outer packaging and slide the contents on to the top shelf of the trolley or onto the tray, taking care not to touch the sterile pack.
- Open the dressing pack using only the corners of the paper, taking care not to touch any of the sterile equipment.
- Place any other required items on the sterile field ensuring the outer packaging does not come into contact with the sterile field.
- Put a pair of non-sterile gloves on to remove any dressings on the patient and ensure that they are positioned appropriately.
- Discard gloves and wash hands.
- Put sterile gloves on.

After
- Dispose of contaminated equipment in the rubbish bag from the dressing pack. Dispose of all packaging.
- Dispose of aprons and gloves in the appropriate waste as per local policy.
- Wash hands.
- Clean the trolley with detergent wipes and dry with a paper towel.

Two-person technique

- An assistant can be very helpful in maintaining the position of the patient, opening packs, and decanting solutions for the person performing the procedure.
- The 'clean practitioner' must wear the sterile gloves and open the first pack to establish a sterile field.
- The second ('dirty') practitioner can then open all the other equipment and drop onto the sterile field.

Clean technique

- This is a modified aseptic technique, aiming to prevent the introduction or spread of micro-organisms and to prevent cross-infection to patients and staff. This is used when true asepsis is not required (e.g. when dealing with contaminated sites or when *removing* drains and catheters).
- Sterile equipment is not always used.
- 'Clean technique' allows the use of tap water, non-sterile gloves, multi-pack dressings, and multi-use containers of creams and ointments.

Box 4.3 ANTT or 'clean' technique?

When to use ANTT

- Insertion, repositioning, or dressing invasive devices such as catheters, drains, and intravenous lines
- Dressing wounds healing by primary intention
- Suturing
- When sterile body areas are to be entered
- If there is tracking to deeper areas or the patient is immunocompromised.

When to use clean technique

- Removing sutures, drains, urethral catheters
- Endotracheal suction, management of tracheostomy site
- Management of enteral feeding lines
- Care of stomas
- Instillation of eye drops.

Box 4.4 Interruptions

- If the sterile procedure is interrupted for more than 30 minutes, new sterile packs should be opened and the sterility process started from scratch.

Subcutaneous and intramuscular injections

Usual sites for subcutaneous injections are upper arms and the abdomen, particularly the periumbilical region.

Intramuscular injections can be administered at any site with adequate muscle mass. Usual sites are deltoids and the gluteal region (upper, outer quadrant of buttock).

Contraindications

- Contraindications regarding the drugs being injected will vary dependent upon the drugs being administered.
- Infection at the injection site.
- Oedema or lymphoedema at the injection site.

Risks

- Incorrect drug and/or dosage administered.
- Allergy to drug(s).
- Haemorrhage, haematoma.
- Infection.
- Injection into a blood vessel.
- Injection into a nerve.

Equipment

- Appropriate syringe.
- 25G (orange) needle (usually).
- Prescribed drug.
- Prescription chart.
- Antiseptic swab.
- Plaster.

Before you start

- Assess patient for drugs required (i.e. for pain relief, vomiting, etc.).
- Refer to prescription chart, double-checking the appropriate drugs and dosage to be given.
  - ▶ Always ensure you are fully aware of any possible side effects of any drugs you are due to administer.
- Double-check the prescription chart for date and appropriate route for administration.
- Check administration of previous dose—not too soon after last dose?
- Ensure that the drug to be given is within its use-by date.
- Check patient and chart for any evidence of allergies, or reactions.
- Once all above completed as per hospital policy, draw-up required drug and check appropriate needle size.
- Complete appropriate documentation.
- Once checked by suitably qualified staff, take drug and prescription chart to the patient.

Subcutaneous procedure

- Introduce yourself, confirm the patient's identity, explain the procedure and obtain informed consent.
- Check with patient: name and date of birth (if capable).
  - If incapable, check name band with another healthcare professional.
- Select appropriate site, and cleanse with the antiseptic wipe.
- Grasp skin firmly between thumb and forefinger of your left hand.
- Insert needle at 45° angle into the pinched skin, then release skin from your grip.
- Draw syringe plunger back, checking for any blood. If none, inject drug slowly.
  - ▶ If any blood is noted on pulling the plunger back, withdraw and stop procedure—provide reassurance and explanation to the patient.
- Once the procedure is completed without complication, withdraw needle and discard into a sharps bin.
- Monitor patient for any negative effects of the drug.

Intramuscular procedure

- Introduce yourself, confirm the patient's identity, explain the procedure, and obtain informed consent.
- Check with patient: name and date of birth (if capable).
  - If incapable, check name band with another healthcare professional
- Select appropriate site, and cleanse with the antiseptic wipe.
  - ❶ If injecting into the buttock, mark a spot at the upper, outer quadrant to avoid the sciatic nerve
  - ❶ If using the deltoid muscle, feel the muscle mass and ensure there is enough muscle to take the needle.
- Insert needle at 90° angle into the skin.
- Draw syringe plunger back, checking for any blood. If none, inject drug slowly.
  - ▶ If any blood is noted on pulling the plunger back, withdraw and stop procedure—provide reassurance and explanation to the patient.
- Once the procedure is completed without complication, withdraw needle and discard into a sharps bin.
- Monitor patient for any negative effects of the drug.

Documentation

- Drugs should always be signed for as per local policy.
- Signature and time should be clearly recorded.
- Site drug administered.
- Reason for drug administration, time given and any impact on the patient should be recorded.
- Immediate vital signs should be recorded in notes.
- Any causes for concern arising from administration of drugs should be clearly documented in the medical notes.
- Signature, printed name, contact details.

Intravenous injections

Intravenous injections can be administered by puncturing the vein with a needle and syringe and injecting directly. The procedure below describes injecting via an intravenous cannula. If no cannula is in place, cannulate first.

▶ Ensure that you comply with the local policy regarding drug administration. In hospital, two healthcare professionals should usually check and administer medication.

Contraindications

- Contraindications regarding the drugs being injected will vary dependent upon the drugs being administered.
- Infection at the cannula insertion site.
- Thrombosis within the vein to be injected.

Risks

- Incorrect drug and/or dosage administered.
- Allergy to drug(s).
- Injection of air embolus.

Equipment

- Appropriate syringe (dependent upon quantity of drug to be administered).
- Prescribed drug.
- Saline flush (10ml syringe with sterile saline).
- Prescription chart.
- Antiseptic swab.

Before you start

- Assess patient for drugs required (i.e. for pain relief, vomiting, etc.).
- ▶ Refer to prescription chart, double-checking the appropriate drugs and dosage to be given.
  - ▶ Always ensure you are fully aware of any possible side effects of any drugs you are due to administer.
- ▶ Double-check the prescription chart for date and appropriate route for administration.
- ▶ Check administration of previous dose—not too soon after last dose?
- ▶ Ensure that the drug to be given is within its use-by date.
- ▶ Check patient and chart for any evidence of allergies, or relevant drug reactions.
- Always comply with the local hand hygiene practices.
- Once all above completed as per hospital policy, draw-up required drug and check appropriate needle size.
- Complete appropriate documentation.
- Once checked by suitably qualified staff take drug and prescription chart to the patient.

Procedure

- Introduce yourself, confirm the patient's identity, explain the procedure and obtain informed consent.
- Check with patient: name and date of birth (if capable).
  - If incapable, check name band with another healthcare professional
  - ❶ The patient may need to be assisted to change position, if unable to move themselves, and to enable access to an appropriate site.
- Cleanse the cannula port with the antiseptic wipe.
- Attach the saline flush to the syringe port and inject a few ml to check patency of the cannula.
  - ▶ Watch for a bleb forming as consequence of extravasation.
- If no problems are encountered, swap the flush for the drug-containing syringe and inject drug slowly.
- To finish, inject a few more ml of saline into the cannula port and re-attach the bung.
- Once the procedure is completed without complication, withdraw needle and discard into a sharps bin.
- Monitor patient for any negative effects of the drug.

Documentation

- Drugs should always be signed for as per local policy.
- Signature and time should be clearly recorded.
- Site drug administered.
- Reason for drug administration, time given, and any impact on the patient should be recorded in the notes.
- Immediate vital signs should be recorded in notes.
- Any causes for concern arising from administration of drugs should be clearly documented in the medical notes.
- Signature, printed name, contact details.

Venepuncture

Risks
- Bleeding, haematoma.
- Infection.
- Accidental arterial puncture.

Inappropriate sites
- Oedematous areas.
- Cellulitis.
- Haematomas.
- Phlebitis or thrombophlebitis.
- Scarred areas.
- Limb in which there is an infusion.
- Upper limb on the side of a previous mastectomy and axillary clearance.
- Limbs with arteriovenous (AV) fistulae or vascular grafts.

Equipment
- Gloves.
- Sterile wipe (e.g. chlorhexidine or isopropyl alcohol).
- Cotton wool balls or gauze.
- Tape.
- Tourniquet.
- Needle (try 12G first).
- Syringe (size depends on amount of blood required).
- Collection bottles.

Procedure: needle and syringe
- Introduce yourself, confirm the patient's identity, explain the procedure, and obtain verbal consent.
- Position the patient appropriately: sat comfortably with arm placed on a pillow.
- Wash hands, put on your gloves and apply the tourniquet proximally.
- Identify the vein; the best location is often at the antecubital fossa.
  • Palpable (not necessarily visible) veins are ideal.
- Clean the site with the wipe, beginning centrally and moving outwards in concentric circles/swirls.
- Whilst the sterilizing solution dries, remove the needle and syringe from packaging and connect together.
- Unsheathe the needle.
- Using your non-dominant thumb, pull the skin taut over the vein in order to anchor it.
- Warn the patient to expect a 'sharp scratch'.
- Insert the needle, bevel up, at an angle of 30 until a flashback is seen within the hub of the needle.
  • With experience you will feel a 'give' as the vein is entered.
- Hold the syringe steady and withdraw the plunger slowly until the required amount of blood is obtained.
- Release the tourniquet.

- Remove the needle, holding cotton wool or gauze to the puncture site.
- Secure the cotton wool or gauze in place or replace with a plaster.
- Vacuum collection bottles are filled by puncturing the rubber top with the needle and allowing the blood to enter the tube.
- Label the tubes at the patient's bedside and dispose of the sharps in a sharps bin.

Procedure: vacuum device

The procedure is much the same as with a syringe but:
- Vacutainer needles are double-ended, with one end a standard needle, the other covered by a rubber sheath. This end inserts into the holder and is screwed in place.
- On penetrating the vein no flashback is seen.
- Once the needle is in place, vacuum collection bottles are inserted into the holder over the sheathed needle in turn—the holder must be held firmly in place.
- Bottles are self-filling; some require filling to a pre-defined level or tests will be invalidated.
- Remove the tourniquet before removing the last bottle, then remove the needle from the skin.

Procedure tips

- If no veins are visible or palpable, don't limit yourself to the upper limb: any peripheral vein will suffice.
  - If veins are still not visible, try warming the limb.
- If several attempts have failed, seek help from a colleague.
- If the vacuum collection system is proving difficult, try using needle and syringe:
  - A 'flashback' will be seen on entering the vein
  - The flow of blood may be controlled
  - If this also proves unsuccessful, try using a butterfly needle (Box 4.5).

Documentation

- Detailed documentation of the procedure is usually not required—but you should record that blood was taken and what tests it has been sent for.
- Record any adverse incidents during the procedure or if multiple attempts were performed.
  - If a particularly good vein was found, you may wish to record this for the benefit of the person taking blood next time.
- Signature, printed name, contact details.

Box 4.5 Butterfly needles

A butterfly is a short needle with flexible 'wings' on either side, and a length of flexible tubing to connect to the syringe. It is easy to manoeuvre once the skin is penetrated, and can be easily fixed in place by the wing, pressed down by the non-dominant thumb. It carries a greater risk of needle-stick injury.

Sampling from a central venous catheter

▶ Central venous lines should only be used for blood sampling if it is not possible to obtain a sample via the peripheral route. Do not risk catheter sepsis or a clotted line unless there are no alternatives.

The following describes venous blood sampling from a line in the internal jugular vein. The principles are the same for a line at any site.

Risks

- Clot or infection in the line.
- Air embolus.
- Physical damage to the line: burst or torn port.

Equipment

- 3 x 10ml syringes.
- 0.9% isotonic or heparinized saline.
- Chlorhexidine spray or iodine solution.
- Sterile gauze.
- Sterile gloves and apron.
- Sterile drape.

Procedure

- Introduce yourself, confirm the identity of the patient, explain the procedure, and obtain verbal consent.
- Stop any infusions (if possible) for at least one minute before sampling.
- Place the patient in a supine position.
- Ask the patient to turn their head away from the line site during the procedure.
- Drape the site and put on a pair of sterile gloves and apron.
- Spray the line end with the chlorhexidine solution or wipe with gauze dipped in iodine.
- Clamp the line port and remove the cap, if present.
- Connect a 10ml syringe to the port and then unclamp.
- Withdraw 5–10ml of blood, clamp the line, and remove the syringe.
- Discard the blood.
- Repeat the procedure with a new syringe, withdrawing 10ml.
- Clamp the line, disconnect the syringe.
  - Keep this sample.
- Fill the final syringe with saline and attach it to the port.
- Unclamp the port and instil the saline.
- Clamp the port again before disconnecting the syringe.
- Replace the port cap.

Procedure tips

- Always be sure to clamp the port *before* removing the syringe and unclamp before withdrawing blood or instilling the saline.
- Most central lines have several ports: which should I use?
  - Blood should ideally be sampled from the port with its hole at the tip of the line—this is often the brown port
  - Check the ports: most will have the gauge printed on them, choose the largest gauge port available.
- Be sure to remove any bubbles from the saline before instilling.
- Infusions must be stopped: otherwise a significant portion of the sample obtained may be the solution that is entering via the other port giving inaccurate results at analysis!

Arterial blood gas sampling

Contraindications
- Negative modified Allen's test.
- Cutaneous or subcutaneous lesion at the puncture site (Box 4.6).
- Surgical shunt (e.g. in a dialysis patient) in the limb.
- Infection or known peripheral vascular disease at the puncture site.
- Coagulopathy.

Risks
- Bleeding.
- Haematoma.
- Arteriospasm.
- Infection.
- False aneurysm formation.
- Arterial occlusion.

Equipment
- Gloves.
- Sterile wipe (e.g. isopropyl alcohol).
- Cotton wool balls.
- Tape.
- Gauze.
- Heparinized self-filling syringe and needle.

Box 4.6 Choosing a site

The radial artery at the level of the radial styloid is the usual site of choice as it is both superficial and easily accessible.

If the vessel is not obviously palpable, it is also possible to sample arterial blood at the brachial artery in the antecubital fossa or femoral artery just distal to the inguinal ligament.

Procedure: radial artery
- Introduce yourself, confirm the patient's identity, explain the procedure, and obtain informed consent.
- Position the patient appropriately: sitting comfortably with arm placed on a pillow, forearm supinated, wrist passively dorsiflexed.
- ▶ Confirm ulnar arterial supply to the hand before starting (modified Allen's test):
  - Compress the radial and ulnar arteries with your thumbs
  - Ask the patient to make a fist and open it
  - The hand should appear blanched
  - Release pressure from the ulnar artery and watch the palm
  - The palm should flush to its normal colour
  - ▶ If not, there may be inadequate ulnar arterial supply and damage to the radial artery during blood taking may result in critical ischaemia.
- Put on your gloves.
- Identify the radial artery with index and middle fingers of your non-dominant hand.

- Clean the site, beginning centrally and spiralling outwards.
- Whilst the sterilizing solution dries, remove the needle and syringe from packaging and attach the needle to the end of the syringe.
- Eject excess heparin from the syringe through the needle.
  - ❶ Check local equipment. Some heparinized syringes contain a heparinized sponge and excess heparin/air should not be expelled
- Warn the patient to expect a 'sharp scratch'.
- Whilst palpating the artery (but not obliterating the pulsation), insert the needle just distal to your fingertips, bevel facing proximally, at an angle of 45–60° until a flashback is seen within the needle chamber.
- Hold the syringe steady and allow it to fill itself with 1–2ml blood.
- As you withdraw the needle, apply the gauze swab to the site, maintaining firm manual pressure over for at least 2 minutes
- Dispose of the needle and apply a vented cap, expelling any excess air.
  - (This may not be necessary depending on your equipment.)

Procedure: brachial artery

- Position the elbow in extension. Angle the needle 60°.

Procedure: femoral artery

- Position the patient with hip extended.
- The pulse is felt 2cm below the midpoint between pubic tubercle and anterior superior iliac spine.
- Angle the needle at 90° to the skin.
- Pressure must be applied for at least 5 minutes.

Procedure tips

- Before you start: know where the analyser is and how to use it!
- The key is carefully palpating the artery and lining the needle up to puncture it. Take your time!
- The majority of the pain comes from puncturing the skin. If no flashback is seen immediately, try repositioning the needle by withdrawing slightly without removing it from the skin.
- If there will be some delay in analysing the sample, store the blood-filled syringe on ice.
- Errors occur: if there is air in the syringe, if the sample is delayed in reaching the analyser (if this is anticipated, put the sample on ice), or if a venous sample is accidentally obtained.

Documentation

- Date, time, indication, consent obtained.
- Record how much (if any) supplemental oxygen the patient is on.
- Artery punctured.
- Modified Allen's test?
- How many passes?
- Any immediate complications.
- Signature, printed name, contact details.

Peripheral venous cannulation

Contraindications

- Cannulae should not be placed unless intravenous access is required.
- Caution in patients with a bleeding diathesis.

Risks

- Infection, which could be local or systemic.

Before you start

- Can the drug be given by another route?
- What is the smallest appropriate cannula? (Table 4.1)
- What is the most appropriate location for the cannula? (Box 4.7)

Box 4.7 Choosing a vein

- Avoid areas of skin damage, erythema, or an arm with an AV fistula
- Excessive hair should be cut with scissors before cleaning the skin
- It is best to avoid joint areas such as the antecubital fossa
  - This can cause kinking of the cannula and discomfort
  - A straight vein, in an area such as the forearm or dorsum of the hand where long bones are available to splint the cannula are usually best.
- Wide-bore access requires siting in large veins and often this is only practicable in the antecubital fossa
- In practice, especially in patients who have been cannulated many times before, it is often necessary to go wherever you find a vein.

Sizing cannulae

- Cannulae are colour-coded according to size. The 'gauge' is inversely proportional to the external diameter.
- The standard size cannula is 'green' or 18G but for most hospital patients, a 'pink' or 20G cannula will suffice. Even blue cannulae are adequate in most circumstances unless fast flows of fluid are required.

Table 4.1 Cannula sizes

Gauge	External diameter (mm)	Length (mm)	Approximate maximum flow rate (ml/min)	Colour
14G	2.1	45	290	Orange
16G	1.7	45	172	Grey
18G	1.3	45	76	Green
20G	1.0	33	54	Pink
22G	0.8	25	25	Blue

Equipment

- Gloves.
- Sterile wipe (e.g. chlorhexidine).
- Cannula of appropriate gauge.
- Sterile saline for injection ('flush') and a 5ml syringe.
- Cannula dressing.
- Cotton wool balls/gauze.
- Tourniquet.

Procedure

- Introduce yourself, confirm the patient's identity, explain the procedure, and obtain informed consent
- Put the gloves on.
- Apply the tourniquet proximally on the limb.
- Once the veins are distended, select an appropriate vein: it should be straight for the length of the cannula.
- Wipe with sterile wipe, beginning where you intend to insert the cannula and moving outwards in circles.
- Fill the syringe with saline and eject any air bubbles.
- Remove the dressing from its packaging.
- Unwrap the cannula and check that all parts disengage easily. Fold the wings down so that they will lie flat on the skin after insertion.
- Using your non-dominant hand, pull the skin taut over the vein in order to anchor it in place.
- Hold the cannula with index and middle fingers in front of the cannula wings, thumb behind the cap.
- Warn the patient to expect a 'sharp scratch'.
- Insert the needle, bevel up, at an angle of 30° to the skin, until a flashback of blood is visible within the chamber of the cannula.
- Advance the needle a small amount further, then advance the cannula into the vein over the needle, whilst keeping the needle stationary.
- Release the tourniquet.
- Place your non-dominant thumb over the tip of the cannula, compressing the vein.
- Flush the cannula with a little saline from the end and replace the cap.
- Write the date on the cannula dressing and secure in place.

Procedure tips

- Local anaesthetic cream may be of benefit if you have time.
- Reliable veins are located on the radial aspect of the wrist (cephalic vein), antecubital fossa, and anterior to the medial malleolus (long saphenous).
- If you fail initially with a large-bore cannula, try a smaller gauge.
- If no veins are visible/palpable at first, try warming the limb in warm water for a couple of minutes.
- It may be useful to get assistance to hold the patient's arm still if they are likely to move it during the procedure.
- If you are unable to cannulate after several attempts, try asking someone else. A pair of fresh eyes make a lot of difference!

Femoral venous catheter insertion

Contraindications
- Fem-fem bypass surgery, IVC filter, infected site, thrombosed vein.

Risks
- Arterial puncture, infection, haematoma, thrombosis, air embolism, arteriovenous fistula, peritoneal puncture.

Equipment
- Central line catheter pack.
  - Containing: central line (16–20cm length, multi-lumen if required), introducer needle, 10ml syringe, guidewire, dilator, blade.
- Large dressing pack including a large sterile drape and gauze.
- Normal saline.
- Local anaesthetic for skin (1% lidocaine).
- Sterile preparation solution (2% chlorhexidine).
- Securing device or stitch.
- Sterile gloves, sterile gown, surgical hat and mask.
- Suitable dressing.

Procedure
- Introduce yourself, confirm the patient's identity, explain the procedure, and obtain written consent if possible.
- Position the patient supine (1 pillow), abduct the leg and place a spill sheet under the patient's leg.
- Identify the entry point: 1–2 cm below the mid-inguinal point and 1cm medial to femoral artery.
- Wearing a surgical hat and mask, wash hands using a surgical scrub technique and put on the sterile gown and gloves.
- Set up a trolley using an aseptic technique:
  - Open the dressing pack onto the trolley creating a sterile field
  - Open the central line catheter pack and place onto the sterile field
  - Flush all lumens of the catheter with saline and clamp the ends
  - Ensure the guidewire is ready for insertion
  - Attach the introducer needle to a 10ml syringe.
- Clean the area with sterile solution and surround with a large drape.
- Inject local anaesthetic into the skin over the entry point.
- Identify the femoral artery with your non-dominant hand.
- Pierce the skin through the entry point with the introducer needle.
- Direct the needle at a 30–45° angle to the skin and aim for the ipsilateral nipple, aspirating as you advance the needle.
- ▶ On hitting the vein the syringe will fill with blood.
- Keeping the needle still, carefully remove the syringe—blood should ooze (and not pulsate) out through the hub of the needle.
- Insert the guidewire part-way through the hub of the needle.
  - Guidewires are over 50cm in length; do not insert more than 20cm.
- Remove the needle over the guidewire ensuring one hand is always holding either the proximal or distal end of the wire.

- Thread the dilator over the wire, firmly pushing it through the skin.
  - This may require a small stab incision in the skin with a blade
  - Aim to get 2–3cm of dilator into the vein, not its full length.
- Check the guidewire has not been kinked by ensuring it moves freely through the dilator.
- Remove the dilator and apply pressure over with gauze to stop oozing.
- Thread the catheter over the guidewire until it emerges through the end of the distal port (unclamp this lumen!).
- Holding the guidewire at its port exit site with one hand, push the catheter through the skin with the other.
- Remove the guidewire.
- Blood should flow out of the end of the catheter.
- Aspirate and flush all ports.
- Fix catheter to skin using either a securing device or stitches.
- Cover with transparent dressing.

Procedure tips

- Placing a sandbag underneath the patient's buttock may improve positioning (if a sandbag is not available, roll up a towel or wrap a 1-litre bag of fluid in a sheet as an alternative).
- Do not force the guidewire. If there is resistance to insertion:
  - Reduce the angle of the needle, attempt a shallower insertion
  - Check you are still within the vein by aspirating with a syringe
  - Rotate the needle: this moves the bevel away from any obstruction.
- ▶ Losing the guidewire can be disastrous—always have one hand holding either the proximal or distal end of it.
- Always consider the possibility of an inadvertent arterial puncture:
  - Signs include pulsatile blood flow, high-pressure blood flow or blood bright red in colour (in the absence of hypotension or hypoxaemia)
  - Do not dilate if in any doubt
  - The use of saline in the aspirating syringe may make flushing the needle easier but also makes it more difficult to differentiate between venous and arterial blood.

Documentation

- Time, date, indication, informed consent obtained.
- Site and side of successful insertion.
- Site, side, and complications of unsuccessful attempt(s).
- Aseptic technique: gloves, gown, hat, mask, sterile solution.
- Local anaesthetic: type and amount infiltrated.
- Technique used: e.g. landmark, ultrasound guidance.
- Catheter used: e.g. triple lumen.
- Length of catheter *in situ* (length at skin).
- Signature, printed name, and contact details.

Central venous access: internal jugular vein

ⓘ This is the 'landmark' technique for the internal jugular vein.

Contraindications

- Infected insertion site.
- Thrombosed vein.
- Coagulopathy.

Risks

- Pneumothorax.
- Arterial puncture.
- Haematoma.
- Air embolism.
- Arrhythmias.
- Thrombosis.
- Arteriovenous fistula.
- Infection.
- Malposition.

Equipment

- Central line catheter pack:
  - Central line (16cm length for right side, 20cm for left side), introducer needle and 10ml syringe, guidewire, dilator, blade.
- Large dressing pack including a large sterile drape and gauze.
- Normal saline.
- Local anaesthetic for skin (1% lidocaine) with suitable (22G) needle and syringe.
- Sterile preparation solution (2% chlorhexidine).
- Sterile gloves, sterile gown, surgical hat and mask.
- Trolley and ECG monitoring.

Procedure

- Introduce yourself, confirm the patient's identity, explain the procedure, and obtain written consent if possible.
- Position the patient supine (1 pillow), tilt the bed head down and place a spill sheet under the patient's head.
- Attach ECG monitoring to the patient.
- Turn the patient's head away from the side of insertion.
- Identify triangle formed by the sternal and clavicular heads of the sternocleidomastoid muscle and the clavicle.
- Identify the entry point at the apex of the triangle.
- Wash hands using a surgical scrub technique and put on the sterile gown and gloves.
- With assistance, set up a trolley using an aseptic technique:
  - Open the dressing pack onto the trolley creating a sterile field
  - Open the central line catheter pack and place onto the sterile field
  - Flush all lumens of the catheter with saline and clamp the ends
  - Attach the introducer needle to a 10ml syringe.

- Clean the area with sterile preparation solution and place a large drape around it.
- Inject local anaesthetic into the skin over the entry point.
- Identify the carotid artery with your non-dominant hand. Pierce the skin through the entry point with the introducer needle ensuring the needle is lateral to the artery.
- Direct the needle at a 30° angle to the skin and advance using continuous aspiration, aiming for the *ipsilateral* nipple.
- On hitting the vein, the syringe will fill with blood.
- Keeping the needle still, carefully remove the syringe.
  - Blood should ooze (not pulsate) through the hub of the needle.
- Insert the guidewire through the needle and watch the ECG.
  - ❶ Guidewires tend to be over 50cm in length but do not introduce more than 20cm as this may lead to arrhythmias.
- Remove the needle over the guidewire ensuring one hand is always holding either the proximal or distal end of the wire.
- Thread the dilator over the wire, firmly pushing it through the skin.
  - This may require a small stab incision in the skin with a blade
  - Aim to get 2–3cm of dilator into the vein, not its full length
- Check the guidewire has not been kinked by ensuring it moves freely through the dilator.
- Remove the dilator over the guidewire and apply pressure over the site with gauze.
- Thread the catheter over the guidewire until it emerges through the end of the distal port (unclamp this lumen!).
  - This may require withdrawing some of the guidewire.
- Holding the guidewire at its port exit site with one hand, push the catheter through the skin with the other.
- ▶ Avoid handling the catheter, in particular its tip.
  - Insert 16cm for a right-sided line and 20cm for a left-sided line.
- Remove the guidewire.
  - Blood should flow out through the end of the catheter.
- Aspirate and flush all ports with normal saline.
- Fix catheter to skin with a fixing device or sutures.
- Cover with a transparent dressing.
- Request a chest radiograph to confirm position.

Documentation

- Time, date, indication, and informed consent obtained.
- Site and side of successful insertion.
- Site, side, and complications of unsuccessful attempt(s).
- Aseptic technique: gloves, gown, hat, mask, type of sterile solution.
- Local anaesthetic: type and amount infiltrated.
- Technique used: e.g. landmark, ultrasound guidance.
- Catheter used: length and number of lumens.
- Aspirated and flushed.
- Length of catheter *in situ* (length at skin).
- Chest radiograph: site of tip, absence/presence of pneumothorax.
- Signature, printed name, and contact details.

Procedure tips

- The right internal jugular vein is usually favoured due to its relatively straight course and the absence of the thoracic duct on this side (Fig. 4.1).
- Tilting the bed head down will minimize the risk of air embolism and help distend the veins of the neck.

Getting started

- Asking the patient to sniff or lift their head off the bed will help identify the sternocleidomastoid muscle.
- Asking the patient to perform the Valsalva manoeuvre will distend the veins of the neck and help identify the internal jugular vein.
- For added safety, you may wish to start by using a 21G ('green') hypodermic needle instead of the introducer needle to 'seek' out the vessel using the same technique.
- Check clotting prior to insertion. Aim for INR <1.5 and platelets >50x10^9/L.
- Minimize spillage.

During the procedure

- ▶ The internal jugular vein is relatively superficial and should be encountered within 2–3cm. Do not continue advancing the needle if the vein has not been hit by this point.
- ▶ Do not force the guidewire in. If there is resistance to guidewire insertion:
  - Try lowering the angle of the needle making it more in line with the long axis of the vessel
  - Check you are still within the vein by aspirating with a syringe
  - Try rotating the needle thereby moving the bevel away from any obstruction.
- ▶ Losing the guidewire can be disastrous. Always have one hand holding either the proximal or distal end of it.
- The use of saline in the aspirating syringe may make flushing the needle easier but also makes it more difficult to differentiate between venous and arterial blood.
- ❶ Always consider the possibility of an inadvertent arterial puncture (Box 4.8):
  - Signs include pulsatile blood flow, high-pressure blood flow, or blood bright red in colour (in the absence of hypotension or hypoxaemia)
  - Do not dilate if in any doubt
  - Consider sending blood for a blood gas to confirm venous placement.

Finishing off

- There is an increased incidence of vascular injuries and thrombosis with left-sided catheters mainly because of insufficient catheter depth leading to the tip abutting the lateral wall of the upper SVC. You must ensure left-sided lines are long enough so that their tip lies within the lower part of the SVC.

- On the chest radiograph, confirm catheter position and the absence of a pneumothorax.
- The tip of the catheter should lie at the junction of the superior vena cava and right atrium which is approximately at the level of the carina.

Alternative approaches
- Anterior approach: midpoint of sternal head of sternocleidomastoid aiming towards ipsilateral nipple.
- Posterior approach: posterior border sternocleidomastoid at the crossing of the external jugular vein aiming for the sternal notch.

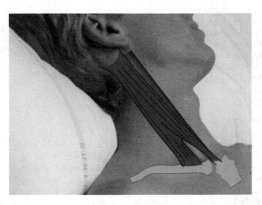

Fig. 4.1 Surface anatomy of the internal jugular vein.

Box 4.8 Structures your needle may hit

In front of the vein
- Internal carotid artery

Behind the vein
- Transverse process of the cervical vertebrae
- Sympathetic chain
- Phrenic nerve
- Dome of pleura
- Thoracic duct on left-hand side.

Medial to vein
- Internal carotid artery
- Cranial nerves IX–XII
- Common carotid and vagus nerve.

Central venous access: subclavian vein

ℹ This is the 'landmark' technique for the right subclavian vein (Fig. 4.2).

Contraindications
- Hyperinflated lungs (e.g. COPD patients).
- Coagulopathy.
- Infected insertion site.
- Thrombosed vein.

Risks
- Pneumothorax.
- Haemorrhage.
- Arterial puncture.
- Air embolism.
- Arrhythmias.
- Thrombosis.
- Arteriovenous fistula.
- Infection.
- Malposition.

Equipment
- Central line catheter pack:
  - Central line (16cm length for right side, 20cm for left side), introducer needle and 10ml syringe, guidewire, dilator, blade.
- Large dressing pack including a large sterile drape and gauze.
- Normal saline.
- Local anaesthetic for skin (1% lidocaine) with (22G) needle and syringe.
- Sterile preparation solution (2% chlorhexidine).
- Sterile gloves, sterile gown, surgical hat and mask.
- Trolley and ECG monitoring.

Procedure
- Introduce yourself, confirm the patient's identity, explain the procedure, and obtain written consent if possible.
- Position the patient supine (1 pillow), place a sandbag between shoulder blades and tilt the bed head down.
- Attach ECG leads onto the patient making sure they are not in the surgical field.
- Turn the patient's head away from the side of insertion.
- Identify the entry point, just inferior to the midpoint of the clavicle.
- Wash hands using a surgical scrub technique and put on the sterile gown and gloves.
- With assistance, set up a trolley using an aseptic technique:
  - Open the dressing pack onto the trolley creating a sterile field
  - Open the central line catheter pack and place onto the sterile field
  - Flush all lumens of the catheter with saline and clamp the ends
  - Ensure the guidewire is ready for insertion
  - Attach the introducer needle to a 10ml syringe.

- Clean the area with sterile preparation solution and place a large drape around it.
- Inject local anaesthetic into the skin over the entry point.
- Insert the introducer needle under the clavicle at a very shallow angle almost parallel to the floor.
- Advance the needle towards the sternal notch, aspirating as you advance.
- On hitting the vein the syringe will fill with blood.
- Keeping the needle still, carefully remove the syringe.
  - Blood should ooze (not pulsate) through the hub of the needle.
- Insert the guidewire through the needle and watch the ECG.
  - ❶ Guidewires tend to be over 50cm in length but do not introduce more than 20cm as this may lead to arrhythmias.
- Remove the needle over the guidewire ensuring one hand is always holding either the proximal or distal end of the wire.
- Thread the dilator over the wire, firmly pushing it through the skin.
  - This may require a small stab incision in the skin with a blade
  - Aim to get 2–3cm of dilator into the vein, not its full length.
- Check the guidewire has not been kinked by ensuring it moves freely through the dilator.
- Remove the dilator over the guidewire and apply gauze to the site to mop up any spills.
- Thread the catheter over the guidewire until it emerges through the end of the distal port (unclamp this lumen!).
  - This may require withdrawing some of the guidewire.
- Holding the guidewire at its port exit site with one hand, push the catheter through the skin with the other.
- ▶ Avoid handling the catheter, in particular its tip.
  - Insert 16cm for a right-sided line and 20cm for a left-sided line
- Remove the guidewire.
  - Blood should flow out through the end of the catheter.
- Aspirate and flush all ports with normal saline.
- Fix catheter to skin with a fixing device or sutures.
- Cover with a transparent dressing.
- Request a chest radiograph to confirm catheter position and the absence of a pneumothorax.

Documentation

- Time, date, indication, and informed consent obtained.
- Site and side of successful insertion.
- Site, side, and complications of unsuccessful attempt(s).
- Aseptic technique: gloves, gown, hat, mask, type of sterile solution.
- Local anaesthetic: type and amount infiltrated.
- Technique used: e.g. landmark, ultrasound guidance.
- Catheter used: length and number of lumens.
- Aspirated and flushed.
- Length of catheter *in situ* (length at skin).
- CXR: site of tip, absence/presence of a pneumothorax.
- Signature, printed name, and contact details.

Procedure tips

Getting started

- Check clotting prior to insertion. Aim for INR <1.5, platelets >50x10^9/L.
- ⚠ Direct pressure cannot be applied on the subclavian vessels so this route should be avoided in patients with a coagulopathy
- ⚠ There is a greater risk of pneumothorax than with internal jugular cannulation. A subclavian approach should, therefore, be avoided in patients with hyperinflated lungs.
- Minimize spillage.
- The underside of the clavicle can be reached by first directing the needle onto the clavicle and then carefully walking off it. The angle of the needle should however remain parallel to the floor.
- Asking an assistant to pull the ipsilateral arm caudally can improve access.
- If a sandbag is not available, roll up a towel or wrap a 1-litre bag of fluid in a spill sheet as an alternative.

During the procedure

- ▶ The subclavian vein should be encountered within 3–4cm. Do not continue advancing the needle if the vein has not been hit by this point.
- ▶ Do not force the guidewire in. If there is resistance to guidewire insertion:
  - Try lowering the angle of the needle making it more in line with the length of the vessel
  - Check you are still within the vein by aspirating with a syringe
  - Try rotating the needle thereby moving the bevel away from any obstruction.
- Catheter malposition, particularly into the ipsilateral internal jugular vein, is more common using the subclavian vein approach.
  - Many guidewires have a 'J' tip. Directing the 'J' tip caudally may help correct placement.
- ▶ Losing the guidewire can be disastrous. Always have one hand holding either the proximal or distal end of it.
- ⚠ Always consider the possibility of an inadvertent arterial puncture (Box 4.9):
  - Signs include pulsatile blood flow, high pressure blood flow or blood bright red in colour (in the absence of hypotension or hypoxaemia)
  - Do not dilate if in any doubt.
- The use of saline in the aspirating syringe may make flushing the needle easier but also makes it more difficult to differentiate between venous and arterial blood.

Finishing off

- The incidence of vascular injuries and thrombosis is increased with left-sided catheters mainly due to insufficient catheter depth leading to the tip abutting the lateral wall of the upper SVC.
  - You must ensure left-sided lines are long enough so that their tip lies within the lower part of the SVC.

- On the chest radiograph, confirm catheter position and the absence of a pneumothorax.
  - The tip of the catheter should lie at the junction of the superior vena cava and right atrium which is approximately at the level of the carina.

Alternative approaches
- Medial approach: junction of medial and middle thirds of the clavicle.
- Lateral approach: lateral to the mid-clavicular point. Often used with ultrasound guidance.

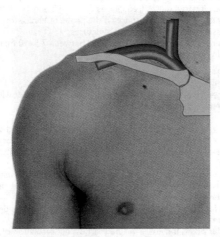

Fig. 4.2 Surface anatomy of the right subclavian vein.

Box 4.9 Structures your needle may hit

In front of the vein
- Clavicle
- Subclavius muscle.

Behind the vein
- Phrenic nerve
- Anterior scalene muscle
- Subclavian artery.

Below vein
- First rib
- Pleura.

Central venous access: ultrasound guidance

▶ Current recommendations in the UK are that ultrasound guidance should be considered when inserting any central venous catheter (NICE guidelines 2002).

Ultrasound basics

- 'Ultrasound' refers to sound waves of such a high frequency as to be inaudible to the human ear (>20 kHz).
- Medical ultrasound uses frequencies between 2 and 14 MHz.
- The 'linear' (straight) transducer is the probe of choice for imaging the vessels and other superficial structures.
- The frequency of the probe should be between 7.5–10 MHz for central venous access.

Basic controls

- Frequency.
  - Higher frequency may result in a better resolution but will not penetrate the tissues as deeply.
- Gain.
  - The gain control alters the amplification of the returned signals
  - This changes the grey scale of the image (can be thought of as increasing the brightness) but may not improve its quality.
- Depth.
  - The depth of the image on screen can be manually adjusted
  - It is wise to see the structures deep to the vessel to be cannulated.
- Focal length.
  - The focal point is usually displayed as an arrow at the side of the image
  - At this point, the image will be sharpest but resolution of the deeper structures will suffer
  - The focal point should be positioned in line with the vein to be cannulated.

Orientation

- By convention, the left of the screen should be that part of the patient to your left (i.e. the patient's right if you are facing the patient, the patient's left if you are scanning from behind them).
  - Touch edge of the probe and watch for the movement on screen to be sure you have the transducer the right way round.

Procedure: internal jugular vein catheterization

- With the patient positioned, squeeze sterile gel onto the patient's neck.
- Hold the probe cover open like a sock. Ask an assistant to squeeze ultrasound gel into the base and *carefully* lower the probe in after it. You can then unfurl the probe cover along the length of the wire using aseptic technique.
- Place probe over the surface markings of the vein (short axis of vessel).
- On the screen, look for two black circles side by side. These represent the vein and the artery.
- Identify the vessels by pressing down with the probe.
  - The vein will be compressible and the artery will not
  - The artery will be pulsatile. ❶ Note that the IJV may also be pulsatile with the patient head down (the JVP)
  - The artery is often circular in cross-section, the vein may be oval or a more complex ovoid shape.
- Follow the course of the vein up the patient's neck and identify a site where the artery sits relatively medial to the vein. At this point, centre the vein on to the screen holding the probe still with your non-dominant hand.
- ❶ Don't press too hard with the probe—you may compress the vein.
- Inject local anaesthetic into the skin around the midpoint of the probe using your dominant hand.
- Insert the introducer needle through the skin at the midpoint of the probe.
- Gently move the needle in and out to help locate the tip and its course on the screen.
  - ❶ The tip of the needle will only be visualized if it is advancing in the same plane as the ultrasound beam.
- Advance the needle (with continuous aspiration) towards the vein ensuring the tip is always in view.
- On hitting the vein, blood will be aspirated into the syringe. Flatten the needle ensuring blood can still be aspirated. At this point, the probe can be removed and the vein be catheterized using the Seldinger technique (see previous pages).
- The ultrasound can be used later in the procedure to ensure that the guidewire lies within the vein, if necessary.

Intravenous infusions

Equipment
- Gloves.
- An appropriate fluid bag.
- Giving set.
- Drip stand.
- 10ml syringe with saline flush.

Procedure
- ❗ Intravenous infusions require intravenous access.
- Check the fluid in the bag and fluid prescription chart.
- Ask a colleague to double-check the prescription and the fluid and sign their name on the chart.
- ❗ Flush the patient's cannula with a few millilitres of saline to ensure there is no obstruction. If there is evidence of a blockage, swelling at the cannula site, or if the patient experiences pain, you may need to replace the cannula.
- Open the fluid bag and giving set, which come in sterile packaging
- Unwind the giving set and close the adjustable valve.
- Remove the sterile cover from the bag outlet and from the sharp end of the giving set.
- Using quite a lot of force, push the giving set end into the bag outlet.
- Invert the bag and hang on a suitable drip-stand.
- Squeeze the drip chamber to half fill it with fluid.
- Partially open the valve to allow the drip to run, and watch fluid run through to the end (it might be best to hold the free end over a sink in case of spills).
- If bubbles appear, try tapping or flicking the tube.
- Once the giving set is filled with liquid, connect it to the cannula.
- Adjust the valve and watch the drips in the chamber.
- Adjust the drip rate according to the prescription (Box 4.10).

Documentation
- Ensure fluid and/or the drug is clearly timed and signed for as per local policy.
- Nursing and/or medical notes should be completed to include the reason for the infusion.
- Medical notes should be used to record any causes for concern arising from administration of the infusion.
- Cannula site (and cannula documentation) should be dated and signed on insertion.
- Ensure any fluid-monitoring chart is complete and updated as appropriate.
- Ensure that all entries in notes finish with your signature, printed name, and contact details.

Box 4.10 Drip rate

- Most infusions tend to be given with electronic devices which pump the fluid in at the prescribed rate. However, it is still important that healthcare professionals are able to set up a drip at the correct flow rate manually
- Using a standard giving set, clear fluids will form drips of about 0.05ml—that is, there will be approximately 20 drips/ml. You can then calculate the number of drips per minute for a given infusion rate as in Table 4.2.

Table 4.2 Drip rate

Prescription Number of hours per litre of fluid	Infusion rate (ml/hour)	Infusion rate (ml/minute)	Drip rate (drips/minute)
1	1000	16	320
2	500	8	160
4	250	4	80
6	166	3	60
8	125	2	40
10	100	1.6	32
12	83	1.4	28
24	42	0.7	14

Arterial line insertion

The following is the procedure for cannulating the radial artery.

Contraindications

- Infection at insertion site.
- Working arterio-venous fistula in the same limb.
- Traumatic injury proximal to the insertion site.
- Vascular insufficiency in the distribution of the artery to be cannulated.
- Significant clotting abnormalities.

Risks

- *Non-vascular:* superficial bleeding, infection, inadvertent arterial injection.
- *Vascular:* vasospasm, thrombosis, thromboembolism, air embolism, blood vessel injury, distal ischaemia.

Equipment

- Arterial catheter set:
  - Arterial catheter (20G), needle, guidewire
- Sterile gloves, sterile gown (+/− surgical hat and mask).
- Dressing pack including a sterile drape.
- Sterile preparation solution (e.g. 2% chlorhexidine).
- Local anaesthetic (e.g. 1% lidocaine), 22G needle, and 5ml syringe.
- (Optional) A three-way tap with a short extension (flushed with normal saline) connected to a 10ml syringe containing normal saline.
- Suture.
- Transducer set with pressurized bag of heparinized saline.

Procedure (modified Seldinger technique)

- Introduce yourself, confirm the patient's identity, explain the procedure, and obtain informed consent.
- Choose a site for arterial line insertion.
- Position the forearm so that it is supported from underneath and hyperextend the wrist.
- Set up a trolley keeping everything sterile:
  - Open the dressing pack onto the trolley creating a sterile field
  - Open the arterial catheter set and place onto the sterile field.
- Wash hands using a surgical scrub technique and put on the sterile gown and gloves.
- Clean the wrist, hand, and forearm with a sterile preparation solution and create a sterile field with the drape.
- Palpate the radial artery with your non-dominant hand and infiltrate the skin overlying the pulsation with some local anaesthetic.
- Insert the arterial needle, directing it towards the radial pulsation at a 30–45° angle. (Do not attach to a syringe.)
  - You can also use a syringe with the plunger removed. This allows identification of the arterial pulsation without excess spillage.
- On hitting the artery, blood will spurt out of the hub of the needle.

- Keeping the needle still, insert the guidewire through the hub of the needle. ❶ Don't force the guidewire.
- Remove the needle leaving the guidewire in place.
- Thread the arterial catheter over the guidewire making sure that the guidewire is seen at all times through the distal end of the catheter.
- Holding the distal end of the guidewire with one hand, push the arterial catheter through the skin with the other.
- Remove the guidewire.
  - Blood should spill out of the end of the catheter if it is within the artery.
- Connect to the short extension of the three-way tap, aspirate and flush with normal saline, and close off the tap.
  - Alternatively, connect immediately to a pressurized transducer set, aspirate and flush
  - ❶ Do not delay connection to transducer and flush-bag
  - ❶ Take extreme care not to allow any air bubbles to flush into the artery (risk of distal embolization).
- Suture in place.
- Label catheter as arterial and inform relevant staff.

Documentation

- Time, date, indication, and informed consent obtained.
- Site and side of successful insertion.
- Site, side, and complications of unsuccessful attempt(s).
- Aseptic technique: gloves, gown, hat, mask, sterile solution.
- Local anaesthetic: type and amount infiltrated.
- Technique used: modified Seldinger, cannula over needle.
- Catheter size used: 20G.
- Aspirated and flushed.
- Signature, printed name, and contact details.

Procedure tips

- ❶ Do not force the guidewire. If there is resistance, try lowering the needle to a shallower angle without removing it from the artery.
- ❶ Cover the floor with spill sheets as the procedure can be messy!
- ▶ The modified Allen's test should be used for assessment of the collateral supply to the hand before the radial artery is punctured but may not be completely reliable in predicting ischaemic injury.

Modified Allen's test

- Compress the radial and ulnar arteries at the wrist and ask the patient to clench their fist.
- Ask the patient to open the hand.
- Release pressure over the ulnar artery.
- Watch the palm for return of colour.
  - Return of colour should normally occur in 5–10 seconds.
- ▶ Return of colour taking over 15 seconds suggests an inadequate collateral supply by the ulnar artery and radial artery cannulation should not be performed.

Fine needle aspiration (FNA)

A method for obtaining a cytological sample of a mass lesion. This procedure should only be performed by, or under strict supervision of, an experienced practitioner.

▶ Fine needle aspiration usually takes place in the radiology department and is performed by an experienced radiologist under ultrasound or CT guidance. The following describes the older, 'blind' technique.

Contraindications

- Bleeding diathesis.
- Overlying infection.
- ❶ Adjacent vital structures.
  - Image-guidance should always be used if available.

Risks

- Bleeding.
- Local infection.
- Damage to surrounding structures depending on site e.g. blood vessels, nerves.

Equipment

- Local anaesthetic (e.g. 1% lidocaine).
- Small-gauge (blue) needle and 10ml syringe.
- Sterile pack.
- Cleaning solution (e.g. chlorhexidine).
- Medium-gauge (green) needle.
- 10 or 20ml syringe for aspiration.
- Sterile gloves.

Procedure

- Introduce yourself, confirm the patient's identity, explain the procedure, and obtain informed consent.
- Position the patient according to the biopsy site, allowing easy palpation of the mass.
- Expose appropriately.
- Wash your hands and put on sterile gloves.
- Clean the area with the cleaning solution and apply drapes.
- Instil local anaesthetic to the skin and subcutaneous tissues, withdrawing the plunger prior to each injection to avoid intravenous injection and warning the patient to expect a 'sharp scratch'.
- Immobilize the mass with your non-dominant hand.
- Using your dominant hand, insert the needle through the skin into the lump, maintaining negative pressure on the plunger as you go.
- Once in the lump, the needle may be moved gently back and forth to obtain a greater volume of cells.
- It may be necessary to insert the needle several times to obtain a sufficient sample.
- Do not expect a large amount of material within the syringe! A tiny sample within the needle will usually suffice.

- Remove the needle and send the sample for cytology (you will need to gently expel the sample from the needle into a suitable container).
- Apply a sterile dressing to the site.

Alternative method
- There are two schools of thought in fine needle aspiration.
- Some practitioners use a small (blue) needle without a syringe attached.
  - This is moved in and out very quickly within the mass whilst also applying rotation
  - Capillary action deposits a cellular sample within the needle which can then be gently expelled using an empty syringe.
- This capillary action technique may result in a larger number of intact cells in the resultant sample as the negative pressure created when using a syringe can disrupt cell membranes.

Documentation
- Date and time.
- Indication, informed consent obtained.
- Type and amount of local anaesthetic used.
- Site of puncture.
- Aseptic technique used?
- How many passes?
- Volume and colour of sample obtained.
- Any immediate complications.
- Tests requested on resultant sample.
- Signature, printed name, and contact details.

Procedure tips
- ❗ Radiological guidance should always be used if available.
- Contact the histopathology department in advance to ensure appropriate transport medium is used.
  - It may be possible to arrange immediate analysis, allowing diagnosis and repeat FNA if insufficient cells are obtained.

Lumbar puncture

Contraindications

- Infected skin or subcutis at the site of puncture.
- Coagulopathy or thrombocytopenia.
- Raised intracranial pressure with a differential pressure between the supra- and infra-tentorial compartments such as seen in space-occupying lesions. If in doubt, image first!

Risks

- Post-procedure headache.
- Infection.
- Haemorrhage (epidural, subdural, subarachnoid).
- Dysaesthesia of the lower limbs.
- Cerebral herniation (always check local procedures regarding contraindication to LP and whether to perform CT head first).

Equipment

- Sterile gloves.
- Sterile pack (containing drape, cotton balls, small bowl).
- Antiseptic solution (e.g. iodine).
- Sterile gauze dressing.
- 1 x 25G (orange) needle.
- 1 x 21G (green) needle.
- Spinal needle (usually 22G).
- Lumbar-puncture manometer.
- 3-way tap (may be included in a lumbar puncture 'kit').
- 5–10ml 1% lidocaine.
- 2 x 10ml syringes.
- 3 x sterile collection tubes and one biochemistry tube for glucose measurement.

Procedure

- Introduce yourself, confirm the identity of the patient, explain the procedure, and obtain verbal consent.
- Position the patient lying on their left-hand side with the neck, knees, and hips flexed as much as possible.
  - Ensure that the patient can hold this position comfortably.
- Place a pillow between the patient's knees to prevent the pelvis tilting.
- Label the collection tubes '1', '2', and '3'.
- Identify the iliac crest. The disc space vertically below this (as you are looking) will be ~L3/L4.
- Mark the space between the vertebral spines at this point with a pen.
- Wash hands and put on the sterile gloves.
- Unwrap all equipment and ensure it fits together correctly.
  - It is usually useful to give the 3-way tap a few twists as it can stick.
- Apply the drapes around the area and sterilize with the antiseptic solution and cotton balls in outward-spiral motions.
- Inject the lidocaine (using a 10ml syringe and the orange needle) at the marked site to raise a small wheal.

- Swap the orange needle for the green one and infiltrate the lidocaine deeper.
- Wait for ~1 minute for the anaesthetic to take effect.
- Introduce the spinal needle through the marked site at about 90° to the skin, heading slightly toward the umbilicus.
  - Keep the bevel facing cranially.
- Gently advance the needle to ~5 cm depth.
- A further slight push of the needle should produce a 'give' as the needle enters the subarachnoid space (this takes a little practice to feel).
- Withdraw the stilette from the needle. CSF should begin to drip out.
- Measure the CSF pressure: connect the manometer to the end of the needle via the 3-way tap (the CSF will rise up the manometer allowing you to read off the number).
- Turn the tap such that the CSF within the manometer pours out in a controlled manner and further CSF can drip freely.
- Collect about 5 or 6 drops into each collection tube *in the order in which they have been labelled.*
- Collect a few more drops into the biochemistry tube for glucose measurement.
- Close the tap so that the manometer will measure the pressure at the end of the collection ('closing pressure').
- Remove the needle, tap, and manometer in one action.
- Apply a sterile dressing.
- Send the fluid for analysis.
  - Cell count (bottles 1 and 3)
  - Microscopy, culture, and sensitivities (bottles 1 and 3)
  - Biochemistry: glucose (biochemistry tube), protein (bottle 2).
- Advise the patient to lie flat for ~1 hour and ask nursing staff to check CNS observations (see local guidelines).

Documentation

- Date, time, indication, and informed consent obtained.
- Vertebral level needle inserted.
- Number of passes before CSF obtained.
- Initial ('opening') pressure and final ('closing') pressure.
- Amount and appearance of CSF.
- Tests samples sent for.
- Any immediate complications.
- Signature, printed name, and contact details.

Procedure tips

- Always use the smallest gauge spinal needle available.
  - In some centres, 'pencil-point' needles are used which are associated with a much reduced incidence of post-procedure headache.
- If the needle strikes bone and cannot be advanced, withdraw slightly, re-angle, and advance in a stepwise fashion until the gap is found.
- Lumbar puncture can be performed with the patient sitting, leaning forwards. This is particularly useful if the patient is obese. However, pressure measurements will be erroneous if taken in this position.

Male urethral catheterization

Contraindications
- Urethral/prostatic injury.

Risks
- Urinary tract infection.
- Septicaemia.
- Pain.
- Haematuria.
- Creation of a 'false passage' through prostate.
- Urethral trauma.
- ❗ Beware latex allergy.

Equipment
- Foley catheter (male) of appropriate French, usually 12–14 gauge.
- 10 ml syringe of sterile water.
- Syringe of lidocaine gel 1% (e.g. Instilligel®).
- Catheter bag.
- Sterile gloves.
- Catheter pack containing drape, kidney dish, swabs/cotton balls, and a small dish.
- Sterile water/chlorhexidine sachet.

Procedure
- Introduce yourself, confirm the patient's identity, explain the procedure, and obtain informed consent.
- Position the patient lying supine with the external genitalia uncovered.
  - Uncover from umbilicus to knees.
- Using aseptic technique, unwrap the equipment and pour the chlorhexidine or sterile water into the dish.
- Wash your hands and put on the sterile gloves.
- Tear a hole in the middle of the drape and place it over the genitals so as to allow access to the penis.
- Use your non-dominant hand to hold the penis upright.
- Withdraw the foreskin and clean around the urethral meatus using the water/chlorhexidine and a swab, moving from the centre outwards.
- Instil local anaesthetic via the urethral meatus, with the penis held vertically.
- Wait at least one minute for the anaesthetic to act.
- Place the kidney bowl between the patient's thighs.
- Remove the tip of the plastic sheath containing the catheter, being careful not to touch the catheter itself.
- Insert catheter into urethra, feeding it out of the plastic wrapper as it is advanced.
- Insert the catheter to the 'hilt'.
  - If the catheter will not advance fully, don't force it. Withdraw a little, extend the penis fully, and carefully try again.

- At this point, urine may begin to drain.
  - Let the hub end of the catheter rest in the kidney bowl to catch the inevitable spills.
- Inflate the balloon using sterile water inserted into the catheter side-arm according to the balloon's capacity (written on the cuff of the balloon lumen).
  - ▶ Watch the patient's face and ask them to warn you if they feel pain.
- Once the balloon is inflated, remove the syringe and attach the catheter bag.
- Gently pull the catheter until you feel resistance as the balloon rests against the bladder neck.
- Replace the foreskin (this is essential to prevent paraphimosis).
- Re-dress the patient appropriately.

Documentation

- Date and time.
- Indication, informed consent obtained.
- Size of catheter inserted.
- Aseptic technique used?
- Volume of water used to inflate the balloon.
- Residual volume of urine obtained.
- Foreskin replaced?
- Any immediate complications.
- Signature, printed name, and contact details.

Procedure tips

- Difficulty passing an enlarged prostate is a common problem. Tricks to try to ease the catheter past include:
  - Ensure the catheter is adequately lubricated
  - Try moving the penis to a horizontal position between the patient's legs as prostatic resistance is reached
  - Ask the patient to wiggle his toes
  - Rotate the catheter back and forth as it advances
  - If catheter fails to pass, consider using larger bore catheter (e.g. 16F instead of 14F) as this may prevent coiling in the urethra.
- If urine fails to drain despite the catheter being fully advanced:
  - Palpate the bladder: if palpable, the catheter is inappropriately placed
  - Manual pressure on the bladder may express enough urine from a near-empty bladder to show itself
  - Aspirate with a bladder syringe, or flush with a little sterile saline.
- ▶ If it is impossible to pass the catheter, ask for help.
  - If all else fails, it may be necessary to proceed to suprapubic catheterization.

Female urethral catheterization

Contraindications

- Urethral injury.

Risks

- Urinary tract infection.
- Septicaemia.
- Pain.
- Haematuria.
- Urethral trauma.
- ❶ Beware latex allergy.

Equipment

- Foley catheter (female) of appropriate French, usually 12–14 gauge.
- 10 ml syringe of sterile water.
- Syringe of lidocaine gel 1% (e.g. Instilligel®).
- Catheter bag.
- Sterile gloves.
- Catheter pack: drape, kidney dish, swabs/cotton balls, and a small dish.
- Sterile water/chlorhexidine sachet.

Procedure

- Introduce yourself, confirm the patient's identity, explain the procedure, and obtain informed consent.
- Position the patient with hips externally rotated and knees flexed. Uncover from waist down.
- Using aseptic technique, unwrap the equipment and pour the chlorhexidine or sterile water into the dish.
- Wash your hands and put on the sterile gloves.
- Tear a hole in the middle of the drape and place it over the genitals so as to allow access.
- Use your non-dominant hand to part the labia.
- Clean around the urethral meatus using the water/chlorhexidine and a swab, moving from the centre outwards.
- Instil local anaesthetic via urethral meatus.
  - Wait at least one minute for the anaesthetic to act.
- Place the kidney bowl between the patient's thighs.
- Remove the tip of the plastic sheath containing the catheter, being careful not to touch the catheter itself.
- Insert catheter into urethra, feeding it out of the plastic wrapper as it is advanced.
- Insert the catheter to the 'hilt'.
- At this point, urine may begin to drain. Let the end of the catheter rest in the kidney bowl to catch any spills.
- Inflate the balloon using sterile water inserted into the catheter side-arm according to the balloon's capacity (written on the cuff of the balloon lumen).
- ▶ Watch the patient's face and ask them to warn you if they feel pain.

- Once the balloon is inflated, remove the syringe and attach the catheter bag.
- Gently pull the catheter until you feel resistance as the balloon rests against the bladder neck.
- Re-dress the patient appropriately.

Documentation

- Date and time.
- Indication, informed consent obtained.
- Size of catheter inserted.
- Aseptic technique used?
- Volume of water used to inflate the balloon.
- Residual volume of urine obtained.
- Any immediate complications.
- Signature, printed name, and contact details.

Procedure tips

- Difficulty passing the catheter may be alleviated by slowly rotating the catheter whilst inserting.
- Difficulty seeing the urethral meatus may be overcome by asking the patient to 'bear down'.
- If urine fails to drain despite the catheter being fully advanced:
  - Palpate the bladder: if palpable, the catheter is inappropriately placed
  - Manual pressure on the bladder may express enough urine from a near-empty bladder to show itself
  - Aspirate with a bladder syringe, or flush with a little sterile saline.
- ▶ If it is impossible to pass the catheter, ask for help
  - If all else fails, it may be necessary to proceed to suprapubic catheterization.

Basic airway management

Airway manoeuvres

The following manoeuvres are performed with the patient lying supine and the attender positioned above the head. The aim is to prevent the flaccid tongue from falling back and causing the epiglottis or tongue itself from occluding the airway (Box 4.11 and Fig. 4.3). These can be performed with no equipment.

Before you start
- Get help!
  - A patient with an obstructed airway can rarely be adequately treated by one individual, even if appropriate kit is within reach.

Head tilt
- Place your hands on the forehead and tilt the head backwards, extending the neck.

Chin lift
- Place two fingertips below the mental protuberance of the mandible, with thumb in front.
- Draw the mandible anteriorly.

Box 4.11 The head tilt/chin lift
- Head tilt and chin lift are usually performed together
- ▶ Head tilt and chin lift are not suitable if there is any suspicion of cervical spinal injury
- Jaw thrust alone should be used in this situation.

Jaw thrust
- Place your fingertips behind the angle of the mandible.
- The base of the thenar eminence of each hand should be rested on the cheek bones.
- Use your fingers to pull the mandible anteriorly, whilst using your thumbs to open the mouth.
- If performed with a mask, the thenar eminence may be used to maintain a good seal.

Procedure tips
- After each manoeuvre, check for success.
- It is worth-while practising these skills on resuscitation dummies prior to having to do them in real life!
- Use the above manoeuvres in conjunction with face masks or bag–valve mask ventilation.

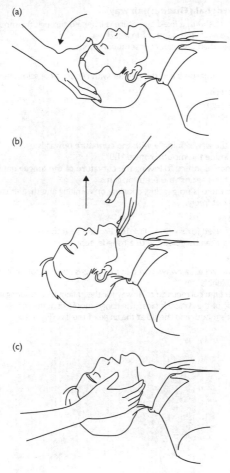

Fig. 4.3 Airway manoeuvres. (a) Head tilt. (b) Chin lift. (c) Jaw thrust.

Oropharyngeal (Guedel) airway

- A stiff tube with a fixed curvature is inserted through the mouth. A flange limits the depth of insertion.
- 🚫 Use when the patient is semi-conscious.

Indications

- Airway compromise in the patient with reduced conscious level.

Contraindications

- Active gag reflex.
- Conscious patient.

Procedure

- Insert the airway initially with the curvature upwards.
- Once inside the mouth, rotate 180°.
- Continue to insert, following the curvature of the tongue until the flange rests against the teeth or gums.
- Ensure there is no gagging, snoring, or vomiting and that air can move in and out freely.

Procedure tips

- May be used for suction (size 10, 12, or 14 catheters).
- Insertion can be guided with a tongue depressor.

Airway sizes

- Oropharyngeal airways come in many sizes and are colour-coded for convenience.
- ▶ Select the correct size of airway for the patient by measuring it against the side of the patient's face. The flange should sit at the corner of the patient's mouth and the tip at the angle of the jaw (Fig. 4.4).

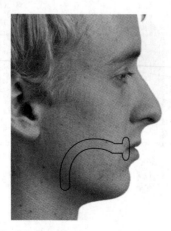

Fig. 4.4 Choose the correct size of oropharyngeal airway by measuring from the corner of the patient's mouth to the angle of the jaw.

Nasopharyngeal airway

- Tolerated better than a Guedel airway in semi-conscious patients.
- Consists of a soft plastic tube with flanged end.
- The pharyngeal end has a bevel and the body is curved to facilitate insertion.
  - Some designs have a small flange and a safety pin is often used to ensure the device does not migrate fully into the patient's nose.

Indications

- Patients with reduced conscious level and/or airway compromise who will not tolerate an oropharyngeal airway (intact gag reflex).

Contraindications

- Known basal skull fracture (relative contraindication).

Procedure

- Lubricate the device.
- Insert bevelled end into the wider nostril.
- Pass the tube along the floor of the nasal airway.
- Aim no higher than the back of the opposite eyeball.
- Use size 10 or 12 catheter for suction if required.
- Advance until the flange is flush against the nostril.

Procedure tips

- If insertion proves difficult, try the opposite nostril.

Airway sizes

- Nasopharyngeal airways come in several sizes, the size is usually stamped on the side.
- Determine the correct size by comparing those available with the pateint's little finger and the distance between the nostril and the tragus (Fig. 4.5).

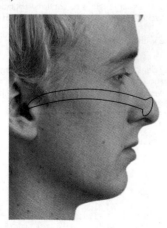

Fig. 4.5 Choose the correct size of nasopharyngeal airway by measuring from the nostril to the tragus.

Laryngeal mask airway (LMA)

- A tube with an inflatable cuff ('mask') around its base to create a seal around the laryngeal inlet.
- ▶ This does not prevent aspiration of stomach contents.

Indications

- Unconscious patient requiring ventilation.

Contraindications

- Conscious patient (absolute).
- Maxillofacial trauma.
- Risk of aspiration.
- >16 weeks' pregnant.

Procedure

- Ensure that the cuff inflates and deflates satisfactorily.
- For insertion, the mask should be completely deflated.
- Deflate the cuff with a 20ml syringe. Lubricate the outer cuff with aqueous gel.
- Gently extend the head and flex the neck (except in possible cervical trauma).
- Hold the LMA tubing near the cuff, like a pen.
- With the mask facing down, pass along the under-surface of the palate until it reaches the posterior pharynx.
- Guide the tube backwards and downwards (using an index finger if necessary) until resistance is felt.
- Remove your hand and fill the mask with the required amount of air (usually 20–30ml).
  - The tube should lift out of the mouth slightly and the larynx is pushed forward if it is in the correct position.
- Connect the bag-valve mask and ventilate.
- Auscultate in both axillary regions to confirm ventilation.
- Insert a bite block/Guedel airway next to the tube in case the patient bites down.
- Secure in place with tape/ribbon.

Procedure tips

- If inadequately deflated, lubricated, or not pressed against the hard palate on insertion, the LMA may fold back on itself making insertion difficult or preventing appropriate positioning of the mask (Fig. 4.6).

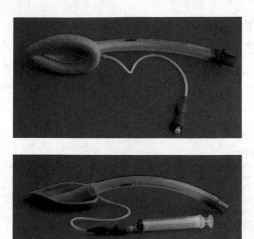

Fig. 4.6 Laryngeal mask airways. (a) Inflated. (b) Deflated.

Oxygen administration

▶ Oxygen is a drug with a correct dosage and side effects which when administered correctly may be life saving.

Oxygen prescribing

The primary responsibility for oxygen prescription at the time of writing lies with the hospital medical staff. It is good practice to record:

- Whether delivery is continuous or intermittent.
- Flow rate/percentage used.
- What SaO_2 should be.

Procedure

- Explain what is happening to the patient and ask their permission.
- Choose an appropriate oxygen delivery device.
- Choose an initial dose:
  - Cardiac or respiratory arrest: 100%
  - Hypoxaemia with $PaCO_2$ < 5.3kPa: 40–60%
  - Hypoxaemia with $PaCO_2$ > 5.3kPa: 24% initially.
- If possible, try to measure a PaO_2 in room air prior to giving supplementary oxygen.
- Apply the oxygen and monitor via oximetry (SaO_2) and/or repeat ABGs (PaO_2) in 30 minutes.
- If hypoxaemia continues, the patient may require respiratory support.

Oxygen administration equipment

- The method of delivery will depend on the type and severity of respiratory failure, breathing pattern, respiratory rate, risk of CO_2 retention, need for humidification, and patient compliance. (Fig. 4.7).
- Each oxygen delivery device comprises an oxygen supply, flow rate, tubing, interface ± humidification.

Nasal cannulae

- These direct oxygen via two short prongs up the nasal passage.
  - Can be used for long periods of time
  - Prevent rebreathing
  - Can be used during eating and talking.
- Local irritation, dermatitis, and nose bleeding may occur and rates of above 4L/min should not be used routinely.

Low flow oxygen masks

- Deliver oxygen concentrations that vary depending on the patient's minute volume. At low flow rates there may be some rebreathing of exhaled gases (they are not sufficiently expelled from the mask).

Fixed performance masks

- A constant O_2 concentration independent of the minute volume.
- The masks contain 'Venturi' barrels where relatively low rates of oxygen are forced through a narrow orifice producing a greater flow rate which draws in a constant proportion of room air through several gaps.

Partial and non-rebreathe masks
- Masks such as this have a 'reservoir' bag that is filled with pure oxygen and depend on a system of valves which prevent mixing of exhaled gases with the incoming oxygen.
- The concentration of oxygen delivered is set by the oxygen flow rate.

High-flow oxygen
- Masks or nasal prongs that generate flows of 50–120L/min using a high flow regulator to entrain air and oxygen at specific concentrations.
- It is highly accurate as delivered flow rates will match a high respiratory rate in patients with respiratory distress. It should always be used with humidification.

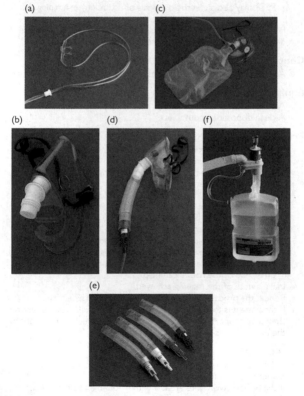

Fig. 4.7 (a) Nasal cannulae. (b) Low flow/variable concentration mask. (c) Non-rebreathe mask. (d) Mask with Venturi valve attached. (e) Selection of Venturi valves. (f) Humidification circuit.

Peak expiratory flow rate (PEFR) measurement

Background
- Normal values vary according to height, age, and gender (Fig. 4.8).
- The value obtained may be compared against this and/or the patient's previous best PEFR.

Indications
- Asthma. Either in an acute attack to assess severity, or during the chronic phase to determine reversibility in response to treatment (>60L/min change defined as reversible).
  - PEFR may also aid in the diagnosis of asthma by examining the greatest variation over two weeks.
- PEFR may also be useful in assessment of COPD, particularly the degree of reversibility in response to inhaled bronchodilator.

Contraindications
- Any features of life-threatening asthma or severe respiratory distress.

Equipment
- A peak flow meter.
- A clean disposable mouthpiece.

Procedure
- Introduce yourself, confirm the patient's identity, explain the procedure, and obtain verbal consent.
- The patient should be standing or sitting upright.
- Ensure that the meter is set to '0'.
- Ask the patient to take a deep breath in, hold the mouthpiece in the mouth, and seal their lips tightly around it.
  - ▶ Ensure that the patient holds the device at the sides, avoiding obstructing the marker with a finger.
- The patient should blow out as *hard* and as *fast* as possible.
  - Patients sometimes have difficulty with this and a quick demonstration or advice to 'imagine blowing out a candle at the other end of the room' can help.
- Make a note of the reading achieved.
- Repeat the procedure and record the best of three efforts.
- If the patient is to keep a record, be sure to explain how to record the readings appropriately. (Sometimes a two-week diary is kept by the patient to assess for diurnal variation.)

Procedure tips
- If the patient is having difficulty performing correctly, a brief demonstration often proves very useful.
- If the highest two values are not within 40L/min, further values should be obtained.

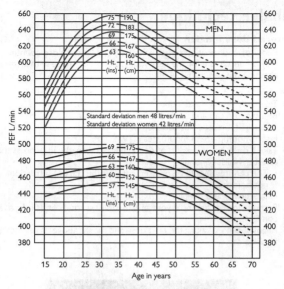

Fig. 4.8 Normal PEFR by age and gender. From BMJ 1989; 298: 1068–70.

Documentation

- Record the highest PEFR in L/min and as a percentage of the patient's best previous or predicted PEFR.
- Make a note of the time and whether the measurement was made before or after therapy.

Inhaler technique

Metered dose inhaler

- Requires coordination to use effectively and lacks a dose counter.
- May be unsuitable for the very young, elderly, or those with arthritis affecting the hands. (Fig. 4.9.)

How to use

- Take only one dose at a time.
- Remove the cap and shake the inhaler several times.
- Sit upright, breathe out completely.
- Insert mouthpiece in mouth, sealing with lips.
- Take a deep breath in. Just after you begin to breathe in depress the canister whilst continuing to inhale.
  - The canister should be pressed *just after* the start of inhalation, not before.
- Inhale slowly and deeply.
- Remove inhaler and hold your breath for 10 seconds or as long as is comfortable.
- Recover before taking the next dose and repeat above as necessary.
- Replace cap.

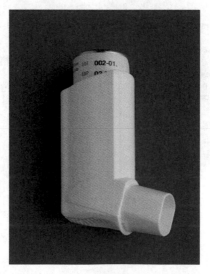

Fig. 4.9 A metered dose inhaler (MDI). A salbutamol inhaler is pictured.

Autohaler

- This is a 'breath-actuated' inhaler, releasing a dose automatically as a breath is taken (Fig. 4.10).
- No hand coordination is required.
- The priming lever, however, can prove difficult to use and requires priming before each dose.

How to use

- Remove cap and shake inhaler several times.
- Prime by pushing the lever into the vertical position whilst keeping the inhaler upright.
- Sit upright, breathe out completely, and insert mouthpiece, sealing with lips.
- Inhale slowly and deeply.
  - Don't stop when the inhaler clicks.
- Remove inhaler and hold your breath for 10 seconds or as long as is comfortable.
- Push lever down and allow time to recover before taking the next dose.
- Once doses are taken, replace cap.

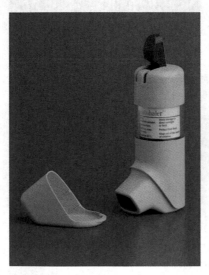

Fig. 4.10 A typical Autohaler.

Procedure tips

- Patients unable to operate the lever by hand may be able to use a hard surface such as the edge of a table for assistance.
- Use inhaler only for the number of doses written on the label.
- Patients should inhale slowly and steadily rather than hard and fast.

Easi-breathe

- Breath-actuated inhaler, as autohaler only primed by opening the cap hence this must be closed and opened again between successive doses (Fig. 4.11).

How to use

- Shake the inhaler several times.
- Hold upright and prime by opening the cap.
- Sit upright, breathe out completely, and insert mouthpiece, sealing with lips.
  - Make sure that your fingers are not covering the air holes at the top.
- Inhale slowly and deeply.
  - ❶ Don't stop when the inhaler puffs.
- Remove inhaler and hold your breath for 10 seconds or as long as is comfortable.
- Close the cap, with the inhaler upright.
- Recover before taking the next dose.

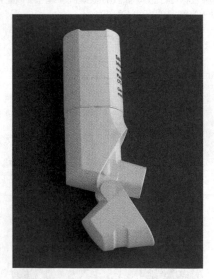

Fig. 4.11 A typical Easi-breathe inhaler.

Procedure tips

- It is essential to close and then open the cap between successive doses. This primes the inhaler.
- Advise the patient not to dismantle the inhaler. Patients used to using MDIs may be tempted to take the top off and attempt to depress the canister manually.

Accuhaler
- Dry powder device, superseding the Diskhaler and Rotahaler (Fig. 4.12).
- Has a dose counter.
- The several step priming mechanism may be difficult for some to manage.

How to use
- Hold the outer casing in one hand whilst pushing the thumb grip away, exposing the mouthpiece, until you hear a click.
- With the mouthpiece towards you, slide the lever away from you until it clicks. The device is now primed.
- Sit upright, breathe out completely, and insert mouthpiece, sealing with lips.
- Inhale quickly and deeply.
  - (In contrast to breath-actuated devices).
- Remove inhaler and hold your breath for 10 seconds or as long as is comfortable.
- To close, pull the thumb grip towards you, hiding the mouthpiece in the cover, until you hear a click.
- Recover before taking the next dose.

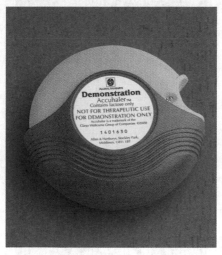

Fig. 4.12 A typical Accuhaler.

Procedure tips
- The Accuhaler must be closed and re-primed between successive doses.
- The dose counter indicates how many doses are left.

Turbohaler

- Dry-powder device with preloaded tasteless drug (Fig. 4.13).
- There is no dose counter, but a window that turns red after 20 doses.
- The device is empty when there is red at the bottom of the window.
- Those with impaired dexterity may find the inhaler difficult to use.

How to use

- Unscrew and remove the white cover.
- Hold the inhaler upright and prime the device by twisting the grip clockwise and anticlockwise as far as it will go (until you hear a click).
- Sit upright, breathe out completely, and insert mouthpiece, sealing with lips.
- Inhale slowly and deeply.
- Remove inhaler and hold your breath for 10 seconds or as long as is comfortable.
- Recover before taking the next dose.
- The device must be primed again between successive doses.

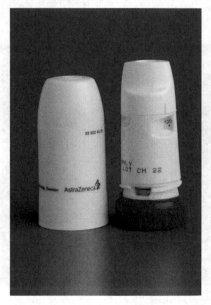

Fig. 4.13 A typical Turbohaler.

Procedure tips

- Advise the patient that they will not feel the dose hit the back of their throat.
- Patients used to an MDI may find this off-putting.

Clickhaler
- Disposable dry-powder inhaler with dose meter which turns red when only 10 doses are left to use.
- The inhaler locks when empty so patients can be sure that they have taken a dose.

How to use
- Take only one dose at a time.
- Remove the cap and shake.
- Whilst holding inhaler upright, depress the button firmly and release until you hear a click.
- Sit upright, breathe out completely, and insert mouthpiece, sealing with lips.
- Inhale deeply.
- Remove inhaler and hold your breath for 10 seconds or as long as is comfortable.
- Recover before taking the next dose and repeat above as necessary.
- Replace cap.

Handihaler
- A dry-powder device with an integrated cap.
- This requires a lower inspiratory flow rate than other devices.
- A dose needs to be inserted via a capsule at each use requiring some dexterity.
- Patients may also find the cap rather hard to open as it requires a moderate amount of strength.

How to use
- Open cap by pulling upwards exposing mouthpiece.
- Open the mouthpiece by pulling upwards exposing the dose chamber.
- Take a capsule from the blister-pack and insert it into the chamber.
- Replace the mouthpiece (it should click shut).
- Press the side button in a few times to pierce the capsule (you can watch through the small window).
- Sit upright, hold head up, and breathe out.
- Seal lips around mouthpiece.
- Breathe in deeply to a full breath.
- Remove inhaler and hold breath for as long as is comfortable.
- Remove the used capsule and replace the cap.

Non-invasive ventilation

▶ Non-invasive ventilation should only be set up by experienced operators. The following is a guide only.

Background
- CPAP = continuous positive airways pressure.
  - CPAP traditionally has its own equipment and 'set-up'
  - Recently more clinicians are delivering CPAP through the BiPAP Vision®. There is also a 'low flow' version used mainly for transport of CPAP dependent patients.
- BiPAP = bilevel positive airways pressure.

Contraindications/cautions
- ▶ Undrained pneumothorax. (Absolute contraindication).
- Facial fractures.
- Life-threatening epistaxis.
- Bullous pulmonary disease.
- Proximal lung tumours (air trapping).
- Active TB (spread).
- Acute head injury.
- Low blood pressure.
- Uncontrolled cardiac arrhythmias.
- Sinus/middle ear infection.

Risks
- Abdominal distension (secondary to 'swallowing' air).
- Decreased cardiac output (drop in BP).
- Pressure sores from mask.
- Aspiration of vomit.
- CO_2 retention if patient breathing small tidal volume against high PEEP.

Documentation
- Oxygen prescription charts.
- Ventilation prescription charts.
- Clear record of ABGs with evidence of time, inspired oxygen, and ventilation levels.
- Good practice to document the 'ceiling' of pressures and FiO_2 for the clinical environment.

CPAP equipment
- Mask (+/− T-piece), hood.
- Head strap (mask), shoulder straps (hood).
- Oxygen circuit and humidification.
- High flow generator (e.g. Whisper Flow®, Vital Signs®).
- PEEP valves (usually 5, 7.5, or 10cmH$_2$O).
- 'Blow off' safety valve (10cmH$_2$O above the PEEP used).

CPAP procedure

- Use available templates to assess appropriate sized interface and minimize air leaks (if using the BiPAP Vision®).
- Decide on level of PEEP to apply.
- Attach PEEP valve to mask (if using traditional set-up, may need T-piece).
- Attach oxygen circuit with humidification including 'blow-off' valve (for safety).
- Set inspired oxygen level.
- Set flow rate to ensure the PEEP valve opens a small distance and never closes.
- Titrate oxygen and PEEP in response to the patient's work of breathing, saturations, pH, PaO_2, and $PaCO_2$.
- If appropriate, set alarms on ventilator (if using BiPAP Vision®).
- Write a prescription chart of PEEP or ventilation settings and acceptable saturations, PaO_2, and $PaCO_2$, continuous or intermittent.

BiPAP equipment

- Interface (face mask, nasal pillows, nasal mask, etc.).
- Head straps.
- Ventilation circuit (exhalation port unless on mask).
- Humidification (if required).
- Ventilator (NIPPY 1/2/3/3+, BiPAP Vision®, etc.).
- Entrained oxygen (unless with ventilator, e.g. BiPAP Vision®).

BiPAP procedure

- Decide on which interface to use.
- Use available templates to assess appropriate sized interface and minimize air leaks.
- Start with low pressures (EPAP 4cmH$_2$O, IPAP 12cmH$_2$O).
  - Slowly increase pressures to levels agreed by MDT, for patient comfort and in response to pH, PaO_2, and $PaCO_2$
  - The aim being to reduce RR and work of breathing, normalize ABGs (for the individual) using the minimal pressures possible.
- Set inspiratory and expiratory times to those of the patient.
- Continually reassess RR as this will change and therefore set times will have to change.
- Titrate oxygen and pressures in response to the patient's saturations, pH, PaO_2, and $PaCO_2$.
- If appropriate set alarms on ventilator.
- Write a prescription chart of ventilation settings and acceptable saturations, PaO_2, and $PaCO_2$.

Pleural fluid aspiration

This describes the procedure for aspirating as much pleural fluid as possible. If only a small sample is required for diagnostic purposes, use a green needle and 20ml syringe and follow a similar method to that described under 'ascitic fluid sampling'. (See Box 4.12 for alternative method.)

▶ Fluid should be aspirated from a position 1–2 intercostal spaces below the highest level at which dullness is percussed.

Contraindications

- Recurrent effusion (chest drain or pleurodesis should be considered).
- Empyema (requires intercostal drainage).
- Mesothelioma (tumour may spread down needle track).
- Bleeding diathesis.

Risks

- Pain.
- Cough.
- Failure to resolve.
- Re-expansion pulmonary oedema.
- Pneumothorax.

Equipment

- Sterile pack.
- Sterile gloves.
- Cleaning solution (e.g. chlorhexidine).
- Large-bore (green) cannula.
- 3-way tap.
- 50ml syringe.
- 5ml 1% lidocaine.
- 23G (blue) needle.
- 2 x 10ml syringe.
- Dressing/gauze.
- Selection of sterile containers and blood bottles.
- Heparinized (ABG) syringe.

Procedure

- Introduce yourself, confirm the patient's identity, explain the procedure, and obtain informed consent.
- Position the patient leaning forward with arms rested on a table or over the back of a chair.
- Percuss the effusion and choose a suitable spot for needle insertion.
- Clean the area with chlorhexidine.
- Using the blue needle and syringe, infiltrate local anaesthetic down to the pleura.
  - ❶ Insert needle *just above* a rib to avoid the neurovascular bundle
  - Be sure to pull back on the syringe each time before injecting to ensure you are not in a blood vessel
  - Once fluid is withdrawn, you have reached the pleura.

- Insert the cannula perpendicular to the chest wall, aspirating with another syringe as you advance until resistance reduces and pleural fluid is aspirated.
- Remove the needle and attach the 3-way tap.
- You may now aspirate fluid using the 50ml syringe.
- Once the syringe is full, close the tap, disconnect the syringe, and empty into a container. Re-attach the syringe, open the tap, and repeat.
  - ❶ The pleural space should never be in continuity with the environment or pneumothorax will occur.
- Do not drain more than 2.5L at one time.
- Remove the cannula and apply the dressing.
- Send samples for:
  - Microbiology: microscopy, culture, Auramine stain, TB culture
  - Chemistry: protein, LDH, pH, glucose, amylase
  - Cytology
  - Immunology: ANA, rheumatoid factor, complement.
- Take simultaneous venous blood for glucose, protein, LDH.
- Request chest radiograph to confirm success and look for iatrogenic pneumothorax.

Procedure tips

- If unsuccessful, aspiration may be performed under ultrasound guidance: discuss with your radiology or respiratory department, depending on local policy.
- Passing a small fluid sample through a blood gas analyser may yield a rapid pH but should be avoided if the sample is purulent.

Documentation

- Date, time, indication, informed consent obtained.
- Aseptic technique used?
- Local anaesthetic used.
- Site needle inserted.
- Colour, consistency, and volume of fluid aspirated.
- Any immediate complications.
- Investigations requested.
- Signature, printed name, and contact details.

Box 4.12 An alternative method

- An alternative method is to attach a fluid-giving set to one port of the 3-way tap and the 50ml syringe to the other
- With this set-up, you can aspirate 50ml into the syringe, turn the tap and empty it down the tubing into a container before turning the tap back to the syringe port
- The syringe, therefore, never needs to be disconnected and the risk of pneumothorax or other complication is reduced.

Pneumothorax aspiration

Simple vs secondary pneumothorax

Simple pneumothorax
- Aspiration is indicated if the rim of pleural air visible on chest radiograph is larger than 2cm or the patient is breathless.
- If initial aspiration is unsuccessful, repeat aspiration may be successful in >30% of cases and may avoid intercostal drain insertion.
- The total volume aspirated should not exceed 2.5L.

Secondary pneumothorax
- That is, a pneumothorax in the presence of underlying lung disease.
- Aspiration is only indicated in minimally symptomatic patients with small pneumothoraces (<2cm) aged <50.

Contraindications
- Previous failed attempts at aspiration.
- Significant secondary pneumothorax.
- Traumatic pneumothorax.

Risks
- Pain.
- Cough.
- Failure to resolve/recurrence.
- Re-expansion pulmonary oedema may theoretically occur if large volumes (>2.5L) are aspirated.

Equipment
- Sterile pack.
- Sterile gloves.
- Cleaning solution (e.g. chlorhexidine).
- Large-bore (green) cannula.
- 3-way tap.
- 50ml syringe.
- 5ml 1% lidocaine.
- 23G (blue) needle.
- 2 x 10mL syringe.
- Dressing/gauze.

Procedure

▶ Pneumothorax is usually aspirated from either 2nd intercostal space at the midclavicular line or the 4th–6th intercostal spaces at the midaxillary line.
- Introduce yourself, confirm the patient's identity, explain the procedure, and obtain informed consent.
- Position the patient leaning back comfortably at about 45°.
- Identify the site for needle insertion and double-check the radiograph to be certain you have the correct side. Confirm with clinical examination.
- Clean the area with the chlorhexidine.

- Infiltrate local anaesthetic down to the pleura using the blue needle and a 10ml syringe.
- Attach the other 10ml syringe to the cannula and insert the cannula perpendicular to the chest wall, aspirating as you advance until resistance reduces.
  - ▶ Insert the cannula *just above* a rib to avoid the neurovascular bundle.
- Remove the needle and quickly attach the 3-way tap and 50ml syringe.
- Aspirate with the syringe; close the 3-way tap when the syringe is full, remove the syringe and eject the air; reattach and open the 3-way tap to continue aspiration.
  - ❶ The pleural space should never be in continuity with the environment (i.e. tap open with syringe detached) or pneumothorax will reaccumulate.
- Aspirate until resistance is felt, or up to a maximum of 2.5L.
- Remove the cannula and apply the dressing.
- Request chest radiograph to re-assess.

Documentation

- Date, time, indication, informed consent obtained.
- Aseptic technique used?
- Local anaesthetic used.
- Site needle inserted.
- Volume of air aspirated.
- Any immediate complications.
- Investigations requested.
- Signature, printed name, and contact details.

Tension pneumothorax

In the case of tension pneumothorax, a wide-bore cannula should be inserted into the 2nd intercostal space, midclavicular line, *without delay* and left open to convert the tension pneumothorax to a simple pneumothorax.

Chest drain insertion (Seldinger)

- This describes the procedure for a Seldinger-type drain. Other drains are available.
- More and more trusts now recommend chest drain insertion under ultrasound guidance. Check your local policy and discuss with your radiology or respiratory departments as appropriate.

Contraindications

- ▶ The need for an emergency thoracotomy. This should not be delayed for the insertion of a chest drain.
- Coagulopathy.
- Large bullae.
- Thoracic/pleural adhesions.
- Skin infection over the insertion site.

Risks

- Inadequate placement.
- Bleeding (local or haemothorax).
- Liver or spleen injury +/− haemoperitoneum.
- Organ penetration (lung, liver, spleen, stomach, colon, heart).
- Infection.
- Iatrogenic pneumothorax.

Equipment

- 10ml 1% lidocaine.
- 10ml syringe.
- 25G (orange) needle.
- 21G (green) needle.
- Sterile gloves.
- Sterile pack (containing cotton balls, drape, container).
- Seldinger chest drain kit.
  - Chest drain, introducer, needle, syringe, scalpel, 3-way tap, wire.
- Suture (e.g. 1.0 Mersilk).
- Cleaning solution (e.g. chlorhexidine or iodine).
- Chest drain tubing and drainage bottle.
- 500ml sterile water.
- Suitable dressing (e.g. Hypofix® or drainfix®).

Procedure

- Introduce yourself, confirm the identity of the patient, explain the procedure, and obtain informed consent.
- ▶ Double-check radiograph and perform clinical examination to be sure of which side needs the drain.
- Position the patient sitting on a chair or the edge of their bed, arms raised and resting on bedside table with a pillow.
- ❶ The usual site for insertion is in the mid-axillary line, within a triangle formed by the diaphragm, the latissimus dorsi, and the pectoralis major ('triangle of safety').
- Mark your spot (just *above* a rib to avoid the neurovascular bundle).

- Wash hands and put on sterile gloves.
- Clean the area with antiseptic solution on cotton wool balls working in a spiral pattern outwards.
- Using the 10ml syringe and orange needle, anaesthetize the skin forming a subcutaneous bleb.
- With the green needle anaesthetize down to the pleura, withdrawing the plunger before injecting each time.
- Use the scalpel to make a small cut in the skin.
- Use the drain-kit needle with the curved tip and syringe (in some kits, this has a central stilette which needs to be removed first). With the curved tip facing downwards (upward for a pneumothorax), advance through the anaesthetized area until you aspirate either air or fluid.
- Remove the syringe and hold the needle steady.
- Thread the guidewire through the needle into the chest.
  - Once the wire is half in the chest, discard the covering.
- Withdraw the needle from the chest but be sure to not remove the guidewire, keeping hold of it at all times, and thread the needle right off the end of the guidewire.
- Thread the introducer over the guidewire and into the chest, twisting back and forth as you go to open up a tract for the drain's passage. Then slide the introducer back off the wire, being careful not to pull the wire out of the chest.
- With the central stiffener in place, thread the drain over the wire and into the chest, curving downwards.
  - Keep hold of the guidewire at all times and do NOT push it into the chest cavity!
- Once the drain is in place, remove the wire and stiffener.
- Attach the 3-way tap, making sure all the ports are closed.
- Stitch the drain in place (unless using a drainfix®).
- Apply a drainfix® or other suitable dressing.
- Attach the drain to the tubing and the tubing to the collection bottle which you have pre-filled with 500ml of sterile water.
- Open the 3-way tap.
  - You should either see the fluid start to flow or air start to bubble in the collection bottle. Ask the patient to take a few breaths and watch the water level in the tubing to see it rising and falling ('swinging').
- Request a post-insertion chest radiograph.

Documentation

- Date, time, indication, informed consent obtained.
- Aseptic technique used?
- Local anaesthetic used.
- Site drain inserted.
- Any immediate complications.
- Colour and consistency of fluid obtained.
- Investigations requested.
- Signature, printed name, and contact details.

Recording a 12-lead ECG

The term '12-lead' relates to the number of directions that the electrical activity is recorded from and is *not* the number of electrical wires attached to the patient!

Equipment

- An ECG machine capable of recording 12 leads.
- 10 ECG leads (4 limb leads, 6 chest leads).
  - These should be attached to the machine.
- Conducting sticky pads ('ECG stickers').

Procedure

- Introduce yourself, confirm the identity of the patient, explain the procedure, and obtain verbal consent.
- Position the patient so that they are sitting or lying comfortably with their upper body, wrists, and ankles exposed.
- Position the stickers on the patient's body (Fig. 4.14).
- The chest leads:
  - V1: 4th intercostal space at the right sternal border
  - V2: 4th intercostal space at the left sternal border
  - V3: midway between V2 and V4
  - V4: 5th intercostal space in the midclavicular line on the left
  - V5: left anterior axillary line, level with V4
  - V6: left mid-axillary line, level with V4.
- The limb leads are often colour-coded:
  - Red: Right arm (Red: Right)
  - Yellow: Left arm (YeLLow: Left)
  - Green: right leg
  - Black: left leg.
- Attach the leads to the appropriate stickers.
- Turn on the ECG machine.
- Ask the patient to lie still and not speak for approximately 10 seconds whilst the machine records.
- Press the button to record, usually marked 'analyse' or 'record'.
- Check the calibration and paper speed:
  - 1mV should cause a vertical deflection of 10mm
  - Paper speed should be 25mm/s (5 large squares per second).
- Ensure the patient's name, date of birth as well as the date and time of the recording are clearly recorded on the trace.
- Remove the leads, discard the sticky electrode pads.

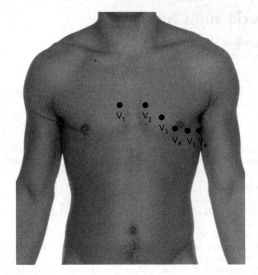

Fig. 4.14 Correct positioning of the chest electrodes for a standard 12-lead ECG.

Procedure tips

- Encourage the patient to relax otherwise muscle contraction will cause interference.
  - If unable to relax, or access to the peripheries is difficult, the 'arm' leads can be placed at the shoulders and the 'leg' leads at the groins.
- Breathing may cause a wandering baseline; breath holding for 6 seconds whilst recording may alleviate this.
- Ensure that you cleanse the area gently with an alcohol swab before attaching an electrode to ensure a good connection.
  - It may be necessary to cut chest hair to allow good contact and adhesion with the chest leads.
- The AC mains electricity may cause interference. If this is the case, try turning off nearby fluorescent lights.

Carotid sinus massage

Background

Anatomy and physiology

- The carotid sinus is located at the bifurcation of the common carotid artery.
  - It lies just under the angle of the jaw at the level of the thyroid cartilage.
- The carotid sinus contains numerous baroreceptors which coordinate homeostatic mechanisms responsible for maintaining blood pressure.
- These baroreceptors are innervated by a branch of the glossopharyngeal nerve (cranial nerve IX), which relays back to the medulla and modulates autonomic control of the heart and blood vessels.

Carotid sinus hypersensitivity

- The carotid sinus can be oversensitive to manual stimulation, a condition known as carotid sinus hypersensitivity (also 'carotid sinus syndrome' or 'carotid sinus syncope').
- In this condition, manual stimulation of the carotid sinus provokes significant changes in heart rate and/or blood pressure due to an exaggerated response to carotid sinus baroreceptor stimulation.
- This may result in marked bradycardia, vasodilation, and subsequent hypotension.
- The patient may complain of episodes of dizziness or syncope related to pressure on the neck (e.g. wearing a tight collar or turning the head quickly).
- The underlying mechanism behind this exaggerated response is not fully understood.

Carotid sinus massage

- Carotid sinus massage is a diagnostic technique used to confirm carotid sinus hypersensitivity and is sometimes useful for determining the underlying rhythm disturbance in supraventricular tachycardia (SVT).
- The procedure acts in a similar way to the Valsalva manoeuvre, increasing vagal tone and, therefore, reducing the heart rate.
- Carotid massage is less effective than pharmaceutical management of SVT (verapamil or adenosine) though is still the preferable choice in the young haemodynamically stable patient.
- ⓘ This procedure should be performed with caution in the elderly as it may cause disruption of atheromatous plaque disease in the carotid artery and result in stroke.

Before you start
- Explain the procedure in full to the patient and obtain written consent.
  - If the test is to confirm carotid sinus hypersensitivity, then warn the patient that they may feel like they are going to faint but reassure them it is a controlled procedure
  - If the test is to determine the underlying rhythm in SVT, explain that they may feel a bit peculiar as the heart rate slows down transiently.
- Auscultate over the carotids for any bruits.
  - ❶ If present the procedure will have to be abandoned as the risk of stroke is significant
- ▶ Document discussion of risks including failure, arrhythmias, stroke, faint, cardiac arrest.
- ▶ Secure intravenous access.
- ▶ Ensure that you have ECG monitoring with a recordable rhythm strip.
- ▶ Ensure access to full resuscitation equipment, including emergency drugs such as atropine and adrenaline.

Procedure
- Position the patient supine on a bed with the neck extended and head turned away from the side to be massaged.
- Whilst watching the ECG monitor (recording on a rhythm strip) gently massage the carotid sinus for 10 to 15 seconds using circular motions of your hand.
- If there is no response, switch to the opposite side.
- If successful (or 'positive' in the case of sinus hypersensitivity), the heart rate will slow.
  - This may allow you to determine the underlying rhythm in SVT.
- Ensure that the patient feels back to normal afterwards.

Documentation
- Date, time, indication, informed consent obtained.
- Intravenous access secured.
- ECG recording equipment operational.
- Emergency drugs on stand-by.
- Insert the rhythm strip into the patient's notes.
- Record details of what was seen on massage.
- Which carotid was used?
- Did the patient feel back to normal afterwards?
- Signature, printed name, and contact details.

Vagal manoeuvres

Background

The purpose

- Vagal manoeuvres can be used to determine the underlying rhythm or terminate supraventricular tachycardia (SVT) in haemodynamically stable patients.
- If the underlying rhythm is atrial flutter, slowing of the ventricular response by increasing vagal tone will reveal flutter waves.
- Vagal manoeuvres are part of the adult peri-arrest algorithm for management of narrow complex tachycardia. They can be performed in a controlled clinical situation (i.e. attached to an ECG machine), or taught to the patient to perform at home if the sensation of the arrhythmia recurs.

Physiology

- Vagal manoeuvres increase vagal tone by activation of the parasympathetic nervous system, conducted to the heart by the vagus nerve.
- Increasing vagal tone impedes the AV node and so slows transmission of the electrical impulse from the atria to the ventricle. In this way, any supraventricular tachycardia that relies upon the AV node will be modified by an increase in vagal tone.

The Valsalva manoeuvre

- This is forced expiration against a closed glottis. Increasing intra-thoracic pressure stimulates baroreceptors in the aortic arch and results in increased vagal stimulation.
- This can be successful in 25–50% of cases.

Procedure

- Ask the patient to take a deep breath in and then 'bear down' as if they are trying to open their bowels (or for women—as if they are in labour).

Some patients may struggle with this concept and so alternatively:

- Give them a 10ml syringe and ask them to blow into the tip, in an attempt to expel the plunger.

The diving reflex

- This involves either submerging the face in ice cold water (not very practical) or covering the face with a towel soaked in ice cold water.

Carotid sinus massage

- This is described separately (see previously).

Eyeball pressure

- ❶ This is not recommended as a clinical procedure as it can be both painful and damaging. Do NOT perform.

Temporary external pacing

🅘 This describes temporary transcutaneous pacing as an emergency.

Before you start

- ▶ External pacing is usually performed in an emergency resuscitation situation following failure of response to initial management as per the bradycardia algorithm (see bradycardia algorithm from Resuscitation Council at 🕮 www.resus.org.uk).
- ▶ A senior doctor should be present and make the decision to proceed with external transcutaneous pacing.
- ▶ There should be a plan in place for an experienced clinician to insert a temporary pacing wire within the next few hours. External pacing should only be a short-term management of decompensated bradycardia.
- ▶ There should also be a bed available for the patient on a high-dependency unit or coronary care unit so that they can be closely monitored by experienced nursing staff whilst waiting for a temporary pacing wire. 🅘 The patient should not be left on a general hospital ward.

Indications

- Symptomatic bradycardia unresponsive to treatment (see bradycardia algorithm from Resuscitation Council at end of this topic).
- Mobitz type II block.
- Complete heart block.
- Heart block secondary to myocardial infarction.
- Profound bradycardia secondary to drug overdose e.g. beta blockers, digoxin.
- Asystole or ventricular standstill.

Overdrive pacing

- External pacing can be used to terminate certain tachyarrhythmias that are unresponsive to initial treatment e.g. polymorphic ventricular tachycardia (torsades de pointes) or refractory ventricular tachycardia.

Risks

- Failure and progression to temporary pacing wire insertion.

Equipment

- Full resuscitation equipment: defibrillator with pacing setting.
- Defibrillator pads.
- Oxygen.
- ECG monitoring.
- Emergency drugs (including atropine and adrenaline).
- Intravenous fluids.
- Sedative drugs (e.g. midazolam or diazepam).
- Analgesia (e.g. morphine).
- Intubation equipment (in case indicated).
- Senior support.

Procedure

- The patient should already have:
  - Large-bore intravenous access
  - Intravenous fluids running (unless in heart failure)
  - Oxygen via a non-rebreathe mask at 15L/min
  - ECG monitor connected and running
  - Interval BP monitoring.
- Place the pacing pads from the defibrillation kit on the patient's chest: one anteriorly in the V3 position and one posteriorly below the left scapula.
- Sedation and analgesia may be required.
- Attach the leads from the defibrillator to the pads.
- Switch the defibrillator to its pacing mode.

Documentation

Temporary external pacing is usually an emergency procedure so documentation may be delayed until the patient is stable. It should outline the resuscitation and external pacing simultaneously:

- Date and time.
- Name and grade of persons present.
- Events leading up to the need for external pacing.
- Any drugs used e.g. atropine or adrenaline, volume/dose, and response.
- Indication for external pacing.
- If patient was conscious, document consent (usually verbal consent only).
- Any sedation used.
- When external pacing commenced.
- Details of plans for temporary pacing wire insertion.
- Sign and bleep/contact details.

DC cardioversion

Indications

- Elective cardioversion of atrial fibrillation.
- Emergency cardioversion in a peri-arrest situation where a tachyarrhythmia is associated with adverse signs.

Equipment

The 'crash trolley' should contain all the equipment required:

- Gloves, aprons, defibrillator, pads, leads, ECG electrodes.
- Oxygen, reservoir bag and mask with tubing, airways.
- Intubation equipment.
- Intravenous fluids, giving sets, selection of syringes, needles, intravenous cannulae, and fixation dressings.
- Access to emergency drugs (atropine, adrenaline, amiodarone).

Contraindications

- Elective: patients unsuitable for general anaesthetic, not anticoagulated or who have not signed a consent form.
- Emergency: only performed when a tachyarrhythmia is associated with adverse events in the presence of a pulse (pulseless rhythms require management as per the resuscitation guidelines).

Risks

- General anaesthetic risk, if performed electively.
- Embolic phenomenon, stroke, myocardial infarction.

Before you start

Elective procedure

- Obtain informed consent and save a copy of signed form.
- Ensure patient fasted >6hrs.
- Check serum potassium (>4.0mmol/L gives greater success).
- Confirm patient anticoagulated for previous 4 weeks (INR >2).
  - Warfarin is continued for 3 months post-procedure if successful.
- The procedure should be performed in an anaesthetic room, following short-acting induction by an anaesthetist.

Emergency procedure

- Ensure a senior doctor is involved in the decision.
- Ensure all other options have been tried or considered.
- If possible discuss with the patient or next of kin.

Energy selection

DC cardioversion usually uses biphasic energies. A reasonable guide is:

- 50 Joules synchronized shock. If fails ...
- 100 Joules synchronized shock. If fails ...
- 150 Joules synchronized shock. If fails ...
- 150 Joules synchronized anteroposterior shock. If fails ...
- ❶ Abandon procedure if elective, consult seniors if emergency (may need ICU input).

Procedure

- Ensure skin is dry, free of excess hair, jewellery is removed.
- Attach the ECG electrodes; red under right clavicle, yellow under left clavicle, green at the umbilicus.
- Switch on defibrillator and confirm the ECG rhythm.
- Place the defibrillator gel pads on the patient's chest; one under the right clavicle and the other inferolateral to the cardiac apex.
- ▶ Select the 'synchronous mode' on the defibrillator.
- ▶ Select the Joules required (see ➋ p.152).
- Place the paddles firmly on the chest on the gel pads.
- Press the charge button on the paddles to charge the defibrillator and shout 'Stand clear! Charging!'
- ▶ Check all persons are standing well clear of the patient and bed (including yourself) and that no-one is touching the patient or bed (including yourself).
- ▶ Ensure the oxygen has been disconnected and removed.
- ▶ Check the monitor again to ensure a shockable rhythm.
- Shout 'Stand clear! Shocking!'.
- Press both discharge buttons on the paddles to discharge the shock.
- Return the paddles to the defibrillator or keep them on the chest if another shock is required.

Documentation

General

- Date, time, and place. Name and grade of persons present.
- ECG rhythm, intravenous access secured.
- Number, volume, dose of any drugs used, and any response noted.
- Type of defibrillator machine used.
- Method of sedation/anaesthetic.
- Asynchronous or synchronous mode. Specify Joules of each shock.
- Confirm rhythm at end and 12-lead ECG findings.
- Sign and bleep/contact details.

Elective

- Indication for DC cardioversion.
- Informed consent obtained (retain copy of signed form).
- State time fasted from.
- Document anticoagulation type and duration.
- Serum potassium level.
- Any drug allergies.
- Name and grade of anaesthetist, type of anaesthetic used.

Emergency

- Events leading up to the peri-arrest situation.
- HR, BP, GCS on arrival and any deterioration.
- Time of decision to shock, name and grade of decision-maker.
- Verbal consent obtained? Type of sedation used.
- Next of kin have been informed or if they are present or en route?

Pericardiocentesis

Contraindications

- Cardiac tamponade secondary to cardiac trauma or aortic dissection (surgical intervention is preferable).
- Recurrent pericardial effusions (surgical pericardial window indicated).

Risks

- Pneumothorax.
- Myocardial perforation.
- Cardiac tamponade.
- Coronary artery laceration.
- Cardiac arrhythmias.
- Intra-abdominal trauma (especially to liver).
- Haemorrhage.
- Infection.
- Acute pulmonary oedema.
- Failure of procedure.
- Death.

Equipment

- Echocardiogram machine and sterile probe cover.
- Pericardial drain kit (14 gauge needle, syringe, guidewire, pigtail catheter, and drain).
- Sterile drape and towels.
- Iodine solution.
- Sterile gloves and gown.
- Local anaesthetic (1% lidocaine).
- 2 x 10ml syringe.
- Orange/blue/green needles.
- Sterile gauze.
- 50ml syringe.
- Three-way tap.
- Suture, scissors, sticky dressing (e.g. Tegaderm®).

You will also need:

- Intravenous access.
- ECG monitoring.
- Access to 'crash' trolley (defibrillator and emergency drugs).

Procedure

- Introduce yourself, explain procedure, and obtain informed written consent.
- Ensure IV access, ECG monitoring, normal clotting, and access to resuscitation equipment.
- (Consider light sedation).
- Position patient supine with 20–30° head tilt.
- Ensure all equipment is sterile and laid out on sterile trolley.
- Wash hands using surgical scrub technique and put on the sterile gown and gloves.

- Clean and drape site at the inferior border of the sternum.
  - Insertion point is below and to the left of the xiphisternum
- ► Confirm location of effusion using echocardiogram machine with sterile probe cover.
- Infiltrate overlying skin and subcutaneous tissue with 1% lidocaine. (Always aspirate before each injection).
- Attach the 10ml syringe attached to the 14G needle.
- Insert the needle between the xiphisternum and left costal margin advancing slowly at 35° to the patient and aiming towards the patient's left shoulder. Aspirate continuously as the needle advances.
  - Pericardial fluid is usually aspirated at about 6–8cm depth
  - Depending on the size of the pericardial effusion and indication for the procedure, you may wish to attach the 50ml syringe and aspirate fluid to send for diagnostic purposes.
- A modified Seldinger technique should be used to insert the drain.
- Once pericardial fluid is aspirated, hold the needle in position, remove the syringe, and insert the guidewire slowly through the needle into the pericardial space.
- Remove the needle, holding the wire in place at all times.
- Pass the catheter over the wire into the pericardial space.
- Once the catheter position is confirmed on echo, remove the wire and attach the three-way tap and drain bag.
- Suture the drain in place and dress to maintain sterility.
- Request a chest radiograph to exclude iatrogenic pneumothorax.

Procedure tips

- ► Pericardiocentesis should be performed by a trained doctor (either cardiologist or thoracic surgeon usually) preferably in a sterile environment (theatre or the cardiac catheterization lab) and under echocardiographic guidance, with access to full resuscitation equipment.
  - ► The only exception is during cardiopulmonary resuscitation when pericardiocentesis is performed as an emergency to exclude cardiac tamponade as a reversible cause of cardiac arrest.
- ► Always check the patient's clotting beforehand.
- The clinician who performed the procedure should confirm the position of the drain using echo.
- Always request a post-procedure chest radiograph to exclude iatrogenic pneumothorax.

Documentation

- Date, time, and place.
- Name and grade of person who performed the procedure (and anyone who supervised).
- Consent obtained (enclose copy of consent form).
- Aseptic technique used and volume of anaesthetic used.
- Approach taken and anatomy confirmed by echocardiogram.
- Any difficulties i.e. 'first pass' or 'second attempt', etc.
- Appearance of pericardial fluid aspirated.
- Volume of pericardial fluid aspirated.

Nasogastric tube insertion

Indications

- Feeding in patients with poor swallow (e.g. post-cerebrovascular accident).
- Lavage of gastric contents in poisoning.
- Post-operative for stomach decompression.
- Bowel obstruction.

Contraindications

- Oesophageal stricture, obstructing tumour.
- Tracheo-oesophageal fistula.
- Achalasia cardia.
- Deviated nasal septum.
- Fractured base of skull.

Risks

- Malpositioning in a lung.
- Trauma to the nasal and/or pharyngeal cavities.
- Perforation of oesophagus.

Equipment

- Lubricant (e.g. Aquagel®).
- pH-testing strips.
- 50 ml syringe.
- Gallipots.
- Dressing pack.
- Nasogastric tube (12–18 French size).
- Hypoallergenic tape.
- Sterile gauze.
- Gloves.
- Disposable bowl.

Procedure

- Introduce yourself, confirm the patient's identity.
- Explain the procedure to the patient, stating that it may be uncomfortable and can cause gagging, which is transient.
- Make sure that the patient understands the procedure and agree a signal to be made if patient wants you to stop (e.g. raising hand).
- To estimate the length of the tube required, measure the distance from the bridge of the nose to the tip of the earlobe and then to the xiphoid process.
- Position the patient semi-upright.
  - If unconscious, place the patient on their side.
- Check the patency of the nostrils and select a suitable side.
- Wash hands and put on gloves.
- Unwrap the tube and lubricate the tip by wiping it through a blob of lubricating gel.
- Insert the tip of the tube in the nostril and advance the tube horizontally along the floor of the nasal cavity backward and downwards.

- As the tube passes into the nasopharynx, ask the patient to swallow if they are able to do so.
  - Using a cup of water and straw often helps here.
- If there is any obstruction felt during advancement, withdraw and try in the other nostril.
- ❗ Watch for any signs of distress; namely cough or cyanosis and remove the tube immediately if any of the above occurs.
- Once the tube has reached the measured distance, secure it in place with the tape.
  - The GOJ is generally 38–42cm from the nostril so advancement of the tube 55–60cm from the nostril usually positions the NG tube tip within the stomach.
- Aspirate a sample of fluid using a syringe.
- Place the aspirate on a pH-testing strip.
  - A pH of 5.5 or less suggests that the tube is in the stomach.
- If no aspirate obtained, change position and try again. If still unsuccessful, perform chest radiography to confirm position.
  - Be sure to leave the internal wire in the tube if you are sending the patient to x-ray. The tube itself is not radio-opaque and will be invisible on the resultant image.
- Once satisfied that the tube lies within the stomach, remove the inner wire and secure the tube to the tip of the nose.
  - It is sometimes helpful to curve the remainder of the tube towards the ear and secure to the cheek also.

Procedure tips

- ❗ Medications such as proton pump inhibitors and acid-suppressing drugs may elevate the pH of the aspirate giving a 'false-negative' result. If in doubt, request a chest radiograph before using.
- ❗ Low-pH fluid may also be aspirated from the lung in cases of aspirated stomach contents. If in doubt, request a chest radiograph before using.
- Chest radiography should be performed routinely in high-risk patients (those that are unconscious, intubated, or have poor swallow).
- The absence of cough reflex does not rule out misplacement of the tube in the airways.
- Auscultation for gurgling in the stomach is not a recommended method for confirming position.

Documentation

- Date, time, indication, informed consent obtained.
- Size of tube inserted.
- Length of tube internally (there are markings on the tube).
- This is important to allow other staff to assess whether the tube has moved in or out since insertion.
- Method by which correct placement was confirmed.
- Any immediate complications.
- Signature, printed name, and contact details.

Ascitic fluid sampling (ascitic tap)

Indications
- Diagnosing nature of new-onset ascites (i.e. exudate or transudate).
- Diagnosis of spontaneous bacterial peritonitis (SBP).
- Cytology to diagnose malignant ascites.

Contraindications
- Acute abdomen that requires surgery.
- Pregnancy.
- Intestinal obstruction.
- Grossly distended urinary bladder.
- Superficial infection (cellulitis) at the potential puncture site.
- Hernia at the potential puncture site.

Risks
- Persistent leak of ascitic fluid.
  - This is more likely if there is a large amount of fluid under tension
- Perforation of hollow viscera (e.g. bowel and bladder). This is very rare.
- Peritonitis.
- Abdominal wall haematoma.
- Bleeding is very rare but may occur if there is injury to inferior epigastric artery (be careful to tap lateral abdominal wall as described).

Equipment
- Sterile gloves.
- Dressing pack.
- Antiseptic solution (e.g. iodine).
- 1% or 2% lidocaine.
- 1 x 20ml syringe.
- 2 x 5ml syringes.
- 21G (green) and 25G (orange) needles.
- Sterile containers.
- Culture bottles.
- Sterile dressing.

Procedure
- Introduce yourself, confirm the patient's identity, explain the procedure, and obtain informed consent.
- Examine the abdomen and select a site for aspiration, three finger-breadths cranial to the anterior superior iliac spine.
  - ▶ Beware of positioning too medial as this risks hitting the inferior epigastric vessels
  - ▶ Be sure to identify and avoid any organomegaly which might interfere with procedure (in patients with massive splenomegaly, for example, avoid left iliac fossa).
- Clean the area with disinfectant and apply sterile drape.
- Using the 25 gauge (orange) needle and the 5ml syringe, administer local anaesthetic to the skin and subcutis, raising a wheal.

- Using the 21 gauge (green) needle, infiltrate deeper tissues, intermittently applying suction until the peritoneal cavity is reached, confirmed by flow of ascitic fluid into the syringe.
- Note the depth needed to enter the peritoneal cavity.
- Discard the used needles and attach a clean 21G needle to the 20ml syringe.
- With the green needle perpendicular to the skin, insert carefully, aspirating continuously until you feel resistance give way.
- Aspirate as much fluid as needed (usually 20ml is plenty).
- Withdraw needle and syringe and apply dressing.
- Send sample for Gram stain and culture (in blood culture bottles), white cell count/neutrophils, biochemistry, cytology (if malignancy suspected).
  - White cell count can be calculated in haematology lab; send fluid in EDTA-containing bottle
  - ▶ Total white cell count >500/mm³ or neutrophils >250/mm³ suggests spontaneous bacterial peritonitis—SBP
  - Neutrophil count is usually a manual procedure via microbiology and may take longer
  - If malignancy is suspected, a large volume of ascites (e.g. 500ml) should be sent to cytology.

Procedure tips

- Check the patient's clotting and platelet count before the procedure and proceed with caution and senior advice if abnormal (correct if platelets <20×10⁹/L, INR ≥2.5).
- Inform the laboratory especially during out of hours if cultures needed urgently and if SBP is suspected.
- ▶ If unable to obtain fluid despite correct technique, do not persist! Stop and seek senior advice.

Documentation

- Date, time, indication, informed consent obtained.
- Type and amount of local anaesthetic used.
- Site aspirated.
- Aseptic technique used?
- How many passes?
- Volume and colour of aspirate obtained.
- Tests requested on samples.
- Any immediate complications.
- Signature, printed name, and contact details.

Abdominal paracentesis (drainage)

The procedure below relates to a 'RocketMedical' non-locking drainage kit—the essence is the same for other catheter kits although minor details may differ. You should refer to the kit's instructions.

Contraindications

- Acute abdomen that requires surgery.
- Pregnancy.
- Intestinal obstruction.
- Grossly distended urinary bladder.
- Superficial infection (cellulitis) at the potential puncture site.
- Hernia at the potential puncture site.
- Caution is needed in the presence of omental or peritoneal metastatic disease. In these cases, drainage is often performed under imaging guidance by a radiologist.

Risks

- Haemodynamic instability, especially in cirrhotic patients; avoided by albumin replacement. (Usually 100ml 20% human albumin solution IV for every 2.5 litres fluid drained—check local protocols with the gastroenterology department).
- Renal dysfunction (in those with abnormal baseline renal function. May need to withhold diuretics and limit drain volume to 5L).
- Wound infection.
- Bleeding.
- Perforation of bowel and bladder.
- Abdominal wall haematoma.

Equipment

- Rocket abdominal catheter pack (catheter sleeve, puncture needle, and adaptor clamp).
- Catheter bag and stand.
- 1 x 25G (orange) needle.
- 1 x 21G (green) needle.
- 3 x 10ml syringes.
- 5ml 1% lidocaine.
- Iodine or antiseptic solution.
- Sterile pack (including gloves, cotton wool balls, and bowl).
- Suitable adhesive dressing.
- Scalpel/blade.

Procedure

- Introduce yourself, confirm the identity of the patient, explain the procedure, and obtain informed consent.
- Ensure that the patient has emptied their bladder.
- Position the patient lying supine or semi-recumbent.
- Percuss the extent of the ascitic dullness.
- Mark your spot in the left iliac fossa within the area of dullness.
  - Double-check clinical examination and imaging, if available. If splenomegaly is present, right-sided drainage is recommended.

- Wash hands and put the sterile gloves on.
- Clean the area thoroughly with antiseptic.
- Infiltrate the skin and subcutaneous tissues with lidocaine via the orange needle and 10ml syringe.
- Attach the green needle to another 10ml syringe and insert into the abdomen, perpendicular to the skin. Advance the needle as you aspirate until fluid is withdrawn.
- Prepare the catheter kit—straighten the curled catheter using the plastic covering sheath provided.
- Take the needle provided in the pack and pass through the sheath such that the needle bevel is directed along inside the curve of the catheter—continue until the needle protrudes from the catheter tip.
- Remove the plastic covering sheath.
- Attach a 10ml syringe to the end of the catheter.
- Make a small incision in the skin using the scalpel.
- Grasp the catheter needle ~10cm above the distal end and, with firm but controlled pressure, push the needle through the abdominal wall to ~3.5–4cm deep, aspirating with the syringe.
- Disengage needle from the catheter hub and advance catheter until the suture disc is flat against the skin, then withdraw the needle.
- Connect adaptor-clamp to the catheter hub and securely attach the rubber portion of the clamp into a standard drainage catheter bag.
- Secure the catheter to the abdomen using a suitable adhesive dressing.
- Ensure the clamp is open to allow fluid to drain.

Procedure tips

- Avoid any scars or engorged veins to minimize complications
- Low-grade coagulopathy is common in cirrhotic patients and fresh frozen plasma and platelets is not routinely recommended; seek advice.
- Fluid leak can be minimized by the z track technique, moving the skin and subcutaneous tissue during insertion of drain, creating a zigzag path.
- If no aspirate is obtained despite multiple attempts, liaise with radiology and request an ultrasound and marking of a suitable site for aspiration. Alternatively, ask the radiology department to insert the drain under ultrasound guidance.

Documentation

- Date, time, indication, informed consent obtained.
- Type and amount of local anaesthetic used.
- Site of drain.
- Aseptic technique used?
- How many passes?
- Volume and colour of fluid obtained.
- Any immediate complications.
- Document the required albumin replacement (if appropriate) and when the catheter should be clamped.
- Signature, printed name, and contact details.

Sengstaken–Blakemore tube insertion

❶ This should be performed only by senior medical staff in close liaison with an anaesthetist and, ideally, with endotracheal intubation especially in agitated patients and those with hepatic encephalopathy.

▶ The threshold to perform endotracheal intubation should be low, as the risk of regurgitation and aspiration is extremely high. Perform nasogastric lavage and stomach evacuation prior to procedure.

Indications

- Life-threatening variceal bleeding where facilities for endoscopy are not available or pending endoscopic therapy.
- Life-threatening variceal bleeding where other modalities to control bleeding have failed.

Contraindications

- Variceal bleeding has ceased or significantly slowed.
- Recent surgery to the gastro-oesophageal junction.
- Known oesophageal stricture(s).

Risks

- Mucosal necrosis due to inadvertent traction.
- Oesophageal perforation. This may be due to a gastric balloon being inflated within the oesophagus or can occur secondary to over- or prolonged-inflation of the oesophageal balloon.
- Aspiration of fluid into the respiratory tract.
- Asphyxiation due to superior migration of the tube and balloons. See last 'procedure tip' below.

Equipment

- Gloves, gown, and goggles.
- Saline flush.
- 2 x 50ml syringe.
- Local anaesthetic spray.
- Sengstaken–Blakemore tube (usually kept in refrigerator to increase its stiffness).
- Lubricant jelly (e.g. Aquagel®).
- Basin with sterile water.
- Suction equipment.
- Sphygmomanometer for pressure monitoring.

Procedure

- Introduce yourself, confirm the patient's identity, explain the procedure to the patient, and obtain informed consent.
- Position the patient at 45 degrees.
- Administer anaesthetic throat spray to the oropharynx.
- Check the balloons in the tube for air leak by inflating them with an air-filled syringe and immersing in a basin of water. Air leak is indicated by air bubbles appearing.
- Deflate the balloons.

- Apply lubricant over the tip of the tube and advance it through the oral cavity slowly until it crosses the gastro-oesophageal junction.
  - The GOJ is generally 38–42cm from the nostril so advancement of the tube 55–60cm usually positions the tip within the stomach.
- Withdraw if the patient becomes breathless.
- Inflate the gastric (**not** oesophageal) balloon with 50ml air.
- At this stage an abdominal radiograph may be performed to confirm the position of the tube in the stomach.
- Once position is confirmed, inflate the gastric balloon to a total volume of 250ml air.
- Pull gently on the tube until resistance is felt.
- Secure with tape near the mouth with gauze pads, maintaining traction and tie the tube to a 500ml bag of saline. A pulley (e.g. a drip stand) is helpful in maintaining traction.
- Mark the tube near the mouth which will serve as an indicator to whether the tube has migrated later.
- Flush the gastric port with normal saline and aspirate at frequent intervals until it is clear, which indicates that bleeding has ceased.
- ⓘ If bleeding continues, inflate the oesophageal balloon with 40ml air and monitor the pressures using the sphygmomanometer frequently.
- ▶ After 12 hours' traction, relax the tension and push the tube into the stomach. If there is evidence of further bleeding, the gastric balloon can be re-inflated and traction re-applied with a view to repeat therapeutic endoscopy.
- ▶ During extubation (usually after 10–12 hours depending on clinical condition), deflate the gastric balloon first then the oesophageal balloon and withdraw the tube slowly.

Procedure tips

- The tube can be used as a measure to control bleeding for about 12–18 hours. It should not be left in place for more than 24 hours.
- Frequent aspirations from the gastric port are needed to assess the status of bleeding.
- The tube has to remain in traction at the gastric balloon which will decompress the varices. However, direct pressure from the tube can cause mucosal ulceration. Examine frequently to ensure that excessive force is not being exerted.
- If the balloons migrate superiorly, airway obstruction may occur. In this instance, as an emergency measure, the tube can be quickly cut with a pair of scissors and removed. Keep a pair of scissors handy.

Documentation

- Date, time, indication, informed consent obtained.
- Those present, including anaesthetic support.
- How many passes?
- Volume balloon inflated to and level of tube insertion.
- Any immediate complications.
- Signature, printed name, and contact details.

Basic interrupted suturing

Many suturing techniques exist. The following is the most commonly used 'interrupted suture'.

Contraindications
- Bites.
- Contaminated wounds.

Risks
- Infection, bleeding, scar (including keloid scars).

Equipment
- Suture (use cutting 3/8 or 1/2 circle needle for skin).
- Needle holder.
- Forceps.
  - Toothed for handling skin; non-toothed for other tissues.
- Scissors.
- Antiseptic solutions, drapes, sterile gloves.
- Dressing.

Procedure: placing the suture
- Introduce yourself, confirm the identity of the patient, explain the procedure, and obtain verbal consent.
- Position the patient comfortably such that the wound is exposed. Clean and drape the area to be sutured.
- Mount the needle in the needle holder approximately 3/4 of the way from the point.
- Start suturing in the middle of the wound to ensure skin edges match up.
- Grasp the skin edge and support it with the forceps.
- Pass the suture through the skin at a 90° vertical angle and approximately 0.5cm from the skin edge.
- Rotate your wrist and follow the contour of the needle until the needle point is visible in the wound.
- Support the needle tip with the forceps and withdraw it from the wound.
- Remount the needle in the needle holder.
- Support the other edge of the wound with the forceps.
- Pass the needle horizontally into the skin edge. Aim to insert the needle at the same depth from the skin's surface as the needle emerged on the other side.
- Rotate your wrist until the needle is seen at the skin surface. Aim to pass the suture 0.5cm from the wound edge.
  - Ensure the entry and exit points are directly opposite each other to prevent distortion of the wound when the suture is tied.
- Support the needle with the forceps and withdraw it through the skin.
- Tie the suture (instructions follow).
- Cut suture ends with scissors leaving 0.5cm behind.
  - This allows it to be grasped when removing.

- Repeat the process proximal and distal to the first suture until the wound is closed.
- Cover with absorbable dressing.
- Give advice on signs of infection, wound care, and when sutures should be removed.

Procedure: tying the suture (instrument tie)

- Pull the suture through until a 2–3cm 'tail' remains.
- Place the needle down at a safe site.
- Grasp the exiting suture (attached to the needle) with your non-dominant hand.
- Hold the needle holders (closed) in your dominant hand.
- Loop the suture twice around the needle holder.
- Without letting the loops slip, open the needle holder and use the tip to grasp the end of the suture 'tail'.
- Move your hands in opposite directions such that the loops slip off the jaws and around the suture.
- Snug the knot down and tighten it.
- Repeat the knot but wrap a single loop around the jaws of the needle holder in the opposite direction to previously.
- Tighten the suture.
- Pull the suture through the wound so the knot lies to one side of wound.
- Repeat until 3 knots are tied.

Documentation

- Date, time, indication, informed consent obtained.
- Anaesthetic used?
- Suture used.
- Number of sutures.
- Dressing.
- Advice given on wound care and follow-up to patient.
- Signature, printed name, and contact details.

Cleaning an open wound

The treatment of open wounds depends on:
- Depth and area.
- Contamination.
- Tissue loss (e.g. vascular, tendon, or nerve damage).
- Other (open fractures or joints, compartment syndrome).

Contraindications
- Major injuries: vascular compromise, tendon rupture, nerve injury, open factures, or joints. These require senior and/or specialist advice.

Risks
- Infection, failure to decontaminate wound.
- Haemorrhage, scar, further surgery.

Equipment
- Anaesthetic (local or general).
- Gloves, mask and eye protection.
- 2 x kidney dish (1 for cleaning solutions, 1 to collect used wash).
- 50ml syringe.
- Swabs.
- Forceps, scalpel, scissors.
- Normal saline or antiseptic solution.
- Sterile drapes.

Procedure

Wound cleaning
- Swab for microbiology if visibly contaminated or history suggestive.
- Clean wound with copious amounts of normal saline and/or water-based antiseptics using syringe.
- Clean wound with swabs from the centre outwards.
  - ▶ Do not use high-pressure irrigation (can push debris deeper).

Inspection and removal of gross contamination
- Photograph wound with adjacent ruler to document size.
- Look for gross contamination and remove with forceps.

Deep palpation
- Methodically check each area visually and with deep palpation to avoid missing contaminants and tissue injuries.
- Use forceps and wound retraction to examine all areas.
- Look for any damage to blood vessel, nerves, and tendons.
- Move the joints above and below the injury whilst looking at the tendon as it moves. Tendon injuries are easily missed if the wound was incurred in a different position to the resting state (e.g. clenched fist).
- ▶ If deep tracts are palpated, the wound may need to be extended into the skin above it to allow adequate drainage.

Excision of dead tissue
- Cut away any dead tissue until healthy tissue is visible.

Maintaining drainage
- Any cavity must be adequately drained.
- Siting a drain:
  - Identify the most dependent part of the cavity
  - Use artery forceps to identify the depth of the tract
  - With scissors, taper and cut a corrugated drain to fit into the tract
  - Pass the tip of the forceps from the tract base so they can be seen at the skin surface
  - Make an incision over the forceps to allow the drain to be sited
  - Grasp the tip of the drain with the forceps and ease into the wound
  - To stop the drain dislodging, a loose suture can be placed into the skin and either around the drain or sutured through one of its corrugations. (This depends on the type of drain used.)
- Finally, wash the wound with antiseptic solution.
- A pack can be used to keep small tracts open and allow drainage.
- A loose suture can be placed to keep the pack in place.
- ▶ Contaminated wounds and bites should not be sutured closed.

Dressing
- A non-stick dressing should be placed over the wound and edges, followed by gauze and bandage or tape.
- Further wound inspection and debridement is required at 48–96 hrs.
  - Examine sooner in heavily contaminated wounds.

Procedure tips
- Instead of a syringe, a normal saline bag and giving set can be used.
- For finger lacerations, a digital nerve block provides good analgesia.
  - 🚫 Don't use adrenaline as this can infarct the digit!
- In an ATLS scenario, open wounds should be photographed and covered with an antiseptic-soaked dressing and bandage. The photograph will allow wound inspection by others, without the need to remove bandages and contaminate the wound further.
- ▶ Always x-ray glass and metal wounds.
- Small superficial wounds with no evidence of contamination on inspection can be closed with interrupted non-absorbable sutures.
  - Patients need to be given information on wound care, signs of infection and when the sutures should be removed.
- Superficial face and head wounds can be closed with skin glue.
- ▶ In some centres, facial wounds are only sutured by maxillo-facial specialists to improve cosmetic results. Check your local policy.

Documentation
- Time, date, mechanism of injury.
- Vaccination status.
- Sensation and pulses.
- Analgesia.
- Draw diagram of wound site and inspection findings.
- How much wash was used?
- If sutured, which suture and when should it be taken out?
- Printed name, signature, and contact details.

Applying a backslab

Plaster backslabs are used as immediate splints for fractures until definitive treatment is performed and are also used to protect the fracture fixation post-surgery.

Equipment
- Stockinette.
- Padding (10cm × 1 roll = above or below elbow backslab, 15cm x 2 rolls = below knee backslab).
- Plaster of Paris bandages.
- Bowl or bucket of water (lukewarm, 25–35°C).
- Crêpe bandage.
- Scissors.

Risks
- Circulatory and nerve impairment, compartment syndrome, pressure sores, joint stiffness.

Procedure tips
- Backslab application is a 2-person procedure.
- Ensure the plaster fits well. A loosely applied cast will not provide adequate splintage and can rub, causing soreness.
- Ensure the plaster does not cause constriction. In the early stages following fractures, the limb may swell, further restricting blood and nervous supply to the limb.
- Ensure bony prominences are adequately padded.

Documentation
- Date, time, indication, informed consent obtained.
- Neurovascular status of limb.
- Procedure performed.
- Plan of further management.
- Patient given instructions to contact staff if develops increasing pain, if extremities change colour (e.g. become blue), or develops 'pins and needles' or numbness.
- Signature, printed name, and contact details.

Procedure: below knee backslab

Used for fractures/dislocations at the ankle and fractures of the foot.

- Use a padded knee rest if available to hold the knee at an angle of 10–15°.
- Hold the ankle at 90° with the foot in a neutral position.
- Cut a length of the stockinette from just below the knee to the toes and apply onto the patient.
- Apply a layer of padding over the stockinette.
  - The padding should extend from just below the knee to the toes
  - Start the padding from one end, rolling it around the limb evenly, overlapping half of the previous turn each time.
- Measure a slab of 10 layers of 15cm plaster of Paris from just below the back of the knee down to the base of the toes.
- Fold the plaster slab and dip it into the water holding the ends.
- Remove the plaster from the water, squeeze gently, and straighten it out.
- Fan out the upper end of the slab to fit the calf area.
- Place from just below the knee along the posterior surface of the lower leg, underneath the heel, and down to the base of the toes.
- Mould and smooth the plaster to fit the contours of the leg with the palms of your hands.
- Cut two side slabs 10x20cm long (length dependent on size of patient) made from 6 layers of plaster.
- Dip these in water and apply either side of the ankle joint.
  - A U-slab may be used instead of the side slabs. A 10cm wide U-slab (made of 6 layers of plaster) should be applied down one side of the leg under the heel of the foot and up the other side. Great care must be taken not to let the slabs overlap anteriorly.
- Finally, turn the stockinette back over the top and bottom edges of the plaster.

Procedure: below elbow backslab

Used for fractures/dislocations at the forearm (including Colles-type injuries) and fractures of the hand.

- Cut a length of the stockinette from just below the elbow to the knuckles, cut a small hole for the thumb.
- Apply the stockinette to the patient.
- Apply a layer of padding over the stockinette.
  - The padding should extend from the elbow to the knuckles of the back of the hand and showing the palmar crease, allowing flexion of the fingers
  - The thumb should be completely free
  - Start the padding from one end, rolling it around the limb evenly and overlapping half of the previous turn each time.
- Cut a length of plaster from below the elbow to the knuckles from a plaster of Paris slab dispenser 15 or 20cm wide (dependent on size of patient), or by forming a slab from 15 or 20cm plaster of Paris bandage using 5 layers.
- Fold the plaster and dip it into the water holding the ends.
- Remove the plaster from the water, squeeze gently, and straighten it out.
- Carefully position the slab on the limb over the padding from just below the elbow, down the dorsal surface of the limb to the knuckles.
- Mould and smooth the plaster to fit the contours of the forearm with the palms of your hands.
- Turn the stockinette back over the edge of the plaster cast at either end.
- Finally, apply the roll of crêpe bandage over the plaster and the overturned stockinette to hold the plaster in place as it sets.

Procedure: above elbow backslab

Used for fractures/dislocations at the forearm and elbow, also supracondy-lar fractures of the humerus.

- Place the limb in a position of 90° flexion at the elbow.
- Cut a length of the stockinette from the axilla to the knuckles of the hand, cut a small hole for the thumb.
- Apply the stockinette to the patient.
- Apply a layer of padding over the stockinette.
  - The padding should extend from the axilla to the knuckles of the back of the hand and showing the palmar crease, allowing finger flexion
  - The thumb should be completely free
  - Start the padding from one end, rolling it around the limb evenly and overlapping half of the previous turn each time.
- Prepare a 10 or 15cm plaster of Paris slab (dependent on patient size), using 5 layers. The slab should be long enough to extend from the axilla to the knuckles of the hand.
- Fold the plaster and dip it into the water holding the ends.
- Remove the plaster from the water, squeeze gently, and straighten it out.
- Carefully position the slab on the limb over the padding running down the posterior surface of the limb over the back of the elbow.
- Mould and smooth the plaster to fit the contours of the forearm with the palms of your hands.
- Prepare two 10cm-wide slabs of five layers of 25cm length (adjust length according to size of patient). Place these on each side of the elbow joint to reinforce it.
- Turn the stockinette back over the edge of the plaster cast at either end.
- Finally, apply the roll of crêpe bandage over the plaster and the overturned stockinette to hold the plaster in place as it sets.

Manual handling

Assisting a patient to stand

Moderate assistance is required from the patient.

Procedure

- ▶ Before beginning the procedure, ensure the patient has been assessed as able to weight-bear.
- ▶ Ensure the immediate area is clutter free.
- Ensure the patient has full understanding of the manoeuvre, and what is expected of them.
- Encourage the patient to move forward in the chair.
- Stand at the side of the chair, slightly behind the patient.
- Ensure the patient, and any other staff, are aware of which command to respond to, e.g. 'ready, steady, stand'.
- With one hand, place your arm nearest the patient around the patient's lower back, reaching as long and as low as is comfortable.
- Place the other hand at the front of the patient's shoulder.
- On the 'stand' command, as the patient rises from the chair, move your position forward such that you are standing next to the patient when upright, to aid their balance.
- ▶ Get the patient to help as much as possible during the manoeuvre e.g. pushing down on the arms of the chair if available.
- ❶ If the patient is unsteady and unable to complete the manoeuvre, gently lower the patient back into the chair and re-assess the situation.

Procedure tips

- ▶ This procedure is only possible with cooperative patients who are able to weight-bear, and are able to understand basic commands.
- This can be carried out with 1 or 2 people, dependent on the patient.
- Allow sufficient time, so that the patient understands the process.
- It is important to encourage the patient's independence; ask them how they would carry out this manoeuvre at home.
- Include the patient in all decision making about the procedure e.g. they may feel comfortable using a Zimmer frame or similar walking aid.
- Check bed area for any furniture/equipment that could be moved to allow more space to complete the manoeuvre.
- ▶ Always check that intravenous fluids, catheters, drains, and other devices are safe and not likely to be pulled out during the procedure.
- Check with staff whether the patient has any history of cognitive problems, violence, or aggression or has any health problems which may prevent or impact upon the manoeuvre.

Documentation

- All patients should have had a moving/handling assessment completed by a physiotherapist in the first 24 hours after admission.
- Any issues raised following the move should be documented in notes.
- Full assessment should be completed prior to each move if the patient's condition has changed.

Assisting a patient to roll whilst lying

Equipment
- 1 (or 2) members of staff.

Procedure
- Ensure the bed/trolley is at waist height and that the brakes are on, to avoid staff injuries.
- ► If the manoeuvre is being carried out with 1 member of staff, always roll the patient towards you.
  - ► If 2 members of staff are available, they should stand either side of the bed/trolley.
- Ensure adequate explanation is given to the patient.
- Ensure the patient's head is facing the way the patient will be moving.
- Place the patient's distant arm across their chest, and flex their distant hip and knee.
- Place an open-palmed hand on the patient's shoulder, and your other hand on the patient's hip or knee.
  - Staff may find it more comfortable to put one of their knees on the bed, to avoid stretching or bending.
- On the command 'ready, steady, roll', move back slightly, aiding the patient to roll towards you.
- Once the patient is on their side, they can be made comfortable with pillows.
- ❶ It is also important to ensure the patient is secure, by making use of bedrails.

Procedure tips
- ❶ Before carrying out the procedure ensure the area around the bed/trolley is clear of any obstacles.
- ❶ Ensure there is adequate space on the bed/trolley for the patient to roll onto.
- It is important to have the correct number of staff available to carry out the manoeuvre.
- Do not rush and leave enough time to explain the procedure to the patient and other members of staff involved.
- It is important to have assessed the patient prior to carrying out this technique, to discover any contraindications to the patient lying on their side (e.g. problems with the patient's head and neck control, or any potential difficulties such as the patient's size).

Documentation
- All patients should have assessments carried out within 24 hours of admission. Care plan to be maintained/consulted as appropriate.
- Any issues or problems with manoeuvre should be documented in the notes.

Assisting a patient to change position in bed (using a glide sheet)

Equipment
- Single-patient use multi-directional slide sheet/glide sheet.
- Minimum of two staff.

Procedure
- Ensure patient is aware of the procedure and has given consent, if able.
- Patient should be lying flat in bed.
- ❶ Discuss desired end position of patient with the other handler(s).
- Move the bed to waist height to prevent staff injuries.
- Ensure the brakes on bed are secure.
- Staff should stand either side of the bed facing each other.
- To place glide sheet under patient, roll patient on bed sheet over to one side of the bed. Either:
  - One staff member leans over patient and pulls the bottom sheet to roll patient onto one side
  - Or, if possible, encourage the patient to roll themselves onto one side.
- The handler nearest the patient should hold sheet (and patient on their side) whilst the glide sheet is inserted by the other handler.
- Place the glide sheet between mattress and bottom sheet.
- The second handler should hold the glide sheet and push as far as possible under bottom sheet and the patient rolls back onto their back.
- Repeat from the other side until glide sheet is fully under the patient.
- Once the sheet is in place, agree which handler will give commands.
- Both handlers should grip the *bed* sheet, with both hands, as close to patient as possible. Place both feet firmly on the floor.
- On command of 'ready, steady, move', both handlers grip bottom sheet and gently move patient to previously agreed position.
- Place pillows appropriately for the patient's revised position.
- Reverse patient movement procedure to remove glide sheet.

Procedure tips
- Do not rush. Ensure sufficient time available to explain the manoeuvre to the patient and safely complete the manoeuvre.
- Check bed area for any furniture/equipment that could be moved to allow more space to complete the manoeuvre.
- ▶ Always check that intravenous fluids, catheters, drains, and other devices are safe and not likely to be pulled out during procedure.
- Check with staff whether the patient has any history of cognitive problems, violence, or aggression or has any health problems which may prevent or impact upon the manoeuvre.
- Ensure bedrails are put back into place following procedure.

Documentation
- All patients should have assessments carried out within 24 hours of admission and placed in their file.
- Any issues or concerns should be documented in the patient's notes to ensure other ward staff are aware of problems.

Transferring a patient laterally using a transfer board

Use to transfer patients who are unable to move themselves.

Equipment

- Patient transfer board or 'Patslide®'.

Procedure

- There should be at least three handlers.
- Open transfer board (if folded) and place on bed/trolley you plan to transfer patient to.
- Explain the manoeuvre to the patient.
- Place destination bed/trolley alongside origin bed/trolley.
  - Ensure there is only a minimal gap between the bed/trolley.
- Check bed is at waist height to prevent staff injuries.
- Staff stand either side of bed/trolley facing each other, two people on the 'destination' side and one on the other.
- ❶ Check brakes on bed and trolley secure.
- Staff at the patient's bedside to lean over patient and grip bed sheet as close to the patient's body as possible in both hands and roll the patient towards them.
- Staff at the bed/trolley onto which patient is to be transferred, put transfer board onto patient's bed/trolley.
- Staff at bedside allow patient to roll back onto board (which should be under the bed sheet).
- On command of 'ready, steady, move'....
- Handlers push and pull patient gently across on transfer board, dependent upon their position.
  - ❶ Staff should ensure their arms remain straight and they do not lean forward, bending at the waist.
- Once patient is transferred, ensure sheets/blankets are replaced.
- Bedrails should be put into place as appropriate.

Procedure tips

- Ensure time is available to safely complete the manoeuvre.
- Check bed area for any furniture/equipment that could be moved.
- Always check IV fluids, catheters, drains, etc. are safe and unlikely to be caught or pulled out during procedure.
- Move any attachments onto transferring bed/trolley prior to the move.
- Check with qualified staff/physiotherapists regarding any changes in the patient's condition prior to manoeuvre.
- Staff should wear suitable footwear and non-restrictive clothing.
- Check with ward staff that patient can be laid flat.
- If NG-fed, ensure it is switched off to prevent patient aspirating.
- ❶ Do not climb onto the bed/trolley.
- ❶ Ensure both surfaces are the same height, making the manoeuvre both easier and more comfortable for the patient.

Documentation

- Any issues or problems with equipment or manoeuvre should be conveyed to the nurse in charge, documented in the notes, and an appropriate incident form completed.

Transferring a patient using a hoist

Limited input from patient. Use this technique to transfer patients who are unable to weight-bear, sit patients up in the bed, or use a bedpan.

Equipment
- Hoist.
- Sling: single patient use (disposable).

Procedure
- ▶ There should be at least two handlers.
  - Check care plan regarding patient's suitability for hoist usage
  - Before getting equipment, ensure manoeuvre is explained to patient.
- Select appropriate sling: small, medium, or large.
- Ensure hoist and sling are compatible.
- Check hoist is able to take patient's weight: most are able to take up to 25 stones (170kg).
- Check bed is at waist height to prevent staff injuries.
- Staff stand either side of bed facing each other.
- 🛑 Check brakes on bed secure.
- Patient should be rolled to one side of bed.
- Lay the hoist sling on the bed.
- Roll the patient to other side of the bed.
  - Sling should now be in a position from patient's head to thigh.
- Place the loops at shoulder end of sling on arm of hoist.
- Pass the thigh-end loops through each other, then place on hoist.
  - ▶ Ensure the loops are correctly positioned before moving.
- One handler should now manage the controls of the hoist.
- Second handler lowers patient's bed, then moves behind the patient/hoist, ready to guide them into the chair.
- Move patient back with hoist.
- Second handler gently guides patient into the chair.
- Once patient is in chair, disconnect loops from hoist.
- Remove sling from beneath lower legs of patient.

Procedure tips
- Ensure sufficient time available to safely complete the manoeuvre.
- Check bed area for any furniture/equipment that could be moved.
- Always check items such as IV fluids, catheters, and drains are safe and unlikely to be caught in hoist or pulled out during procedure.
- Check with qualified staff/physiotherapists regarding any changes in the patient's condition prior to manoeuvre. Transfer may be inadvisable.
- Staff should wear suitable footwear and non-restrictive clothing.
- Hoist should only be used to transfer patients short distances.
- Ensure hoist is fully charged before commencing manoeuvre.
- 🛑 Ensure the brakes of the hoist are 'off'. This will allow the hoist to find its own centre of gravity.

Documentation
- Any issues with equipment or manoeuvre—advise nurse in charge and document in notes and complete an appropriate incident form.

Transferring a patient using a log roll

Use this technique to transfer patients in whom a cervical spine injury is suspected or confirmed. The following assumes that the patient's neck is immobilized in a brace or blocks.

Equipment
- ▶ Minimum five members of staff.
- Patient transfer board or 'Patslide®'.

Procedure
- ▶ The most senior member of the team should take charge of the patient's head and neck and initiate commands.
- Ensure adequate explanation is given to the patient, and to all members of staff involved.
- Place destination bed alongside origin bed at waist height.
- One member of staff should position themselves at the head end of the patient, the other three should be spread alongside the patient, at the origin side. The final member of staff should be at the destination.
- ❶ Check brakes on bed secure.
- ▶ The person responsible for the patient's head should have one hand either side of the patient's head, supporting the patient's shoulders.
- ▶ The person responsible for the patient's upper body should have one hand on the patient's distant shoulder, and the other on the lateral aspect of the patient's chest.
- ▶ The person responsible for the patient's pelvis should have one hand on the lateral aspect of the pelvis and the other under the thigh.
- ▶ The person responsible for the patient's lower legs should have both hands under the calves.
- On the command 'ready, steady, roll' the three members of staff at the side of the patient will slowly move backwards with straight arms, rolling the patient towards them.
- Staff at the bed/trolley onto which patient is to be transferred, put transfer board onto patient's bed/trolley.
- On the command 'ready, steady, roll' the four members of staff at the side of the patient roll the patient back flat, keeping the neck straight.
- One member of staff should now move around the bed such that there are two on each side and one at the head.
- On the command of 'ready, steady, move', handlers move the patient gently across keeping the head and neck immobilized.

Procedure tips
- Ensure sufficient time available to safely complete the manoeuvre.
- Check bed area for any furniture/equipment that could be moved.
- Staff should wear suitable footwear and non-restrictive clothing.
- ▶ It is essential that the patient's body be kept in alignment, and the manoeuvre is carried out in one smooth and controlled movement.

Documentation
- Any issues with equipment or manoeuvre, advise nurse in charge and document in notes and complete an appropriate incident form.

Aiding a falling patient

- ▶ It is essential that if a patient falls, the member of staff **must not** try to catch the patient, but must allow them to fall, as there is no safe method for this situation.
- ▶ Allowing the patient to fall may feel contrary to the staff's natural instincts to help but trying to catch a patient will only result in injury to staff.
- ❶ Instead, every attempt must be made to reduce injury to the patient (e.g. moving objects out of the patient's way if possible).

Falling in a forward direction

- If a member of staff is walking with a patient as they fall in a forward direction, the member of staff must allow the patient to fall.

Falling towards a member of staff

- If the fall is towards the member of staff, it may be possible to control the patient's movements safely to minimize injury to them.
- The member of staff should move close to the patient, standing directly behind them with their leg closest to the patient flexed. Then they should gently guide the patient's body down their flexed leg to the floor.

Procedure tips

- The risk of falling should be minimized by only performing tasks appropriate to the patient's ability (e.g. only allow patients to walk if they are fully mobile).
- Use equipment to reduce the risk of falls i.e. Zimmer frames or walking sticks.
- ❶ A patient falling is an unpredictable and sudden event. However, the member of staff should take every care to maintain a good posture at all times, avoiding twisting or stretching.
- ▶ If present when a patient falls, the member of staff should immediately call for assistance, to ensure an adequate number of staff are present if the situation turns into an emergency.

Documentation

- All patients should have assessments carried out within 24 hours of admission and placed in their file.
- Any fall or issues should be documented in the patient's notes to ensure other ward staff are aware of problems.

Aiding a fallen patient

- ▶ It is important to assess the fallen patient immediately, to establish the cause for the fall and any immediate consequences (e.g. fainting, fractures, or cardiac arrest) so that staff can respond to the situation accordingly.

Equipment
- Minimum of two members of staff.
- Other equipment dependent on circumstances:
  - Two chairs, trolley, slide sheets, hoist with appropriate sling.

Procedure: if patient is cooperative
- Instructions may be given to help the patient up from the floor. Ask the patient to follow this routine:
- Roll onto their side ...
- Push up on their hands until they are in a sitting position ...
- Bend their knees up and move onto all fours ...
- Place their hands onto the seat of a chair for balance ...
- Move one leg forward, so they are in a half-kneeling position ...
- At this point, the patient should be able to push with their hands to stand up, and sit on a chair placed behind them.
- If needed, the patient can now be hoisted onto a trolley for further assessment.

Procedure: if patient is uncooperative
- A hoist should be used.

Procedure: if fallen in a confined space
- Place a slide sheet under their body.
- With a minimum of two members of staff, the patient can then be slid on the floor a short distance to allow better access to assist the patient.
  - It is essential that the members of staff maintain a good posture at all times during this procedure.

Procedure tips
- ▶ It is essential to establish the cause of the fall and act accordingly.
- ▶ It is important that, as the patient is moving up from the floor, their condition is continuously monitored.
  - ❶ If the patient has fainted, they may be at risk of falling again.
- It is important to allow the patient time to carry out the manoeuvre, as this will reduce the amount of manual assistance required from staff.
- ▶ It is extremely important that the patient is NEVER LIFTED.
  - Lifting a patient is hazardous and may result in staff injury.

Clinical data interpretation

Electrocardiography

Other clinical data

Electrocardiography (ECG)

The first step in making sense of an electrocardiogram (ECG) printout is to understand the electrical conduction process in the normal heart.

Electrophysiology of the heart

Cardiac myocytes

In their resting state, the surface of cardiac myocytes (muscle cells) is polarized with a potential difference of 90mV across the cell membrane (negatively charged intracellularly and positively charged extracellularly).

Depolarization (reversal of this charge) results in movement of calcium ions across the cell membranes and subsequent cardiac muscle contraction. It is this change in potential difference that can be detected by the ECG electrodes and represented as deflections on a tracing.

The basics of the tracing

It is easiest to imagine an electrode 'looking' at the heart from where it is attached to the body.

Depolarization of the myocytes that spreads towards the electrode is seen as an upwards deflection, electrical activity moving away from the electrode is seen as a downwards deflection and activity moving to one side but neither towards nor away from the electrode is not seen at all (see Fig. 5.1).

Electrical conduction pathway

In the normal heart, pacemaker cells in the sinoatrial (SA) node initiate depolarization. The depolarization first spreads through the atria and this is seen as a small upward deflection (the 'P' wave) on the ECG.

The atria and the ventricles are electrically isolated from each other. The only way in which the impulse can progress from the atria to the ventricles normally is through the atrioventricular (AV) node. Passage through the AV node slows its progress slightly. This can be seen on ECG as the isoelectric interval between the P wave and QRS complex, the 'PR interval'.

Depolarization then continues down the rapidly conducting Purkinje fibres—bundle of His, then down left and right bundle branches to depolarize both ventricles (see Fig. 5.2). The left bundle has two divisions (fascicles). The narrow QRS complex on ECG shows this rapid ventricular depolarization.

Repolarization of the ventricles is seen as the T wave. Atrial repolarization causes only a very slight deflection which is hidden in the QRS complex and not seen.

▶ The P wave and QRS complex show the electrical depolarization of atrial and ventricular myocardium respectively, but the resultant mechanical muscle contraction—which usually follows—cannot be inferred from the ECG trace (e.g. in pulseless electrical activity (PEA)).

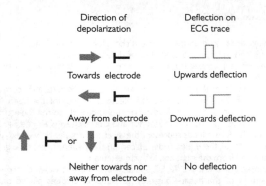

Fig. 5.1 Diagrammatic representation of how waves of depolarization are translated onto the ECG trace depending on the relationship to the electrodes.

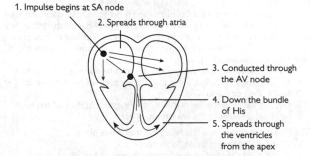

Fig. 5.2 Diagrammatic representation of the electrical conduction pathway in the normal heart.

The 12-lead ECG

Leads

Electrodes are placed on the limbs and chest for a '12-lead' recording. The term '12-lead' relates to the number of directions that the electrical activity is recorded from and is not the number of electrical wires attached to the patient.

The 6 chest leads (V_{1-6}) and 6 limb leads (I, II, III, aVR, aVL, aVF) comprise the 12-lead ECG. These 'look at' the electrical activity of the heart from various directions. The chest leads correspond directly to the 6 electrodes placed at various points on the anterior and lateral chest wall (see Fig. 5.3). However, the 6 limb leads represent the electrical activity as 'viewed' using a combination of the 4 electrodes placed on the patient's limbs—e.g. lead I is generated from the right and left arm electrodes.

▶ Remember there are 12 ECG leads—12 different views of the electrical activity of the heart—but only 10 actual electrodes placed on the patient's body.

❶ Additional leads can be used (e.g. V_{7-9} extending laterally around the chest wall) to look at the heart from further angles such as in suspected posterior myocardial infarction.

ECG orientation

When a wave of myocardial depolarization flows towards a particular lead, the ECG tracing shows an upwards deflection. A downward deflection represents depolarization moving away from that lead. The key to interpreting the 12-lead ECG is therefore to remember the directions at which the different leads view the heart.

The 6 limb leads look at the heart in the coronal plane (see Fig. 5.4).

- aVR looking at the right atrium (all the vectors will be negative for this lead in the normal ECG).
- aVF, II, and III viewing the inferior or diaphragmatic surface of the heart.
- I and aVL examining the left lateral aspect.

The 6 chest leads examine the heart in a transverse plane ...

- V_1 and V_2 looking at the right ventricle.
- V_3 and V_4 at the septum and anterior aspect of the left ventricle.
- V_5 and V_6 at the anterior and lateral aspects of the left ventricle.

Although each of the 12 leads gives a different view of the electrical activity of the heart, for the sake of simplicity when considering the standard ECG trace, we can describe the basic shape common to all leads (see Fig. 5.5).

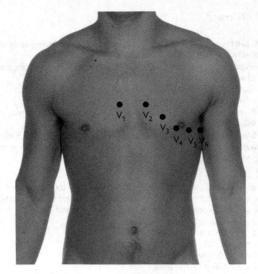

Fig. 5.3 Correct placement of the 6 chest leads.

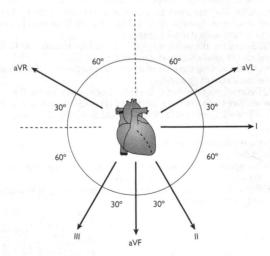

Fig. 5.4 The respective 'views' of the heart of the 6 limb leads. Note the angles between the direction of the limb leads – these become important when calculating the cardiac axis.

The ECG trace

Waves

- P wave represents atrial depolarization and is a positive (upwards) deflection—except in aVR.
- QRS complex represents ventricular depolarization and comprises:
  - Q wave: so called if the first QRS deflection is negative (downwards). Pathological Q waves are seen in myocardial infarction
  - R wave: the first positive (upwards) deflection—may or may not follow a Q wave
  - S wave: a negative (downwards) deflection following the R wave.
- T wave represents ventricular repolarization and is normally a positive (upwards) deflection, concordant with the QRS complex.

Rate

- The heart rate can be calculated by dividing 300 by the number of large squares between each R wave (with machine trace running at the standard speed of 25mm/sec and deflection of 1cm/10mV).
  - 3 large squares between R waves = rate 100
  - 5 large squares = rate 60.
- Normal rate 60–100 beats/minute.
  - Rate <60 = bradycardia
  - Rate >100 = tachycardia.

Intervals and timing

- PR interval: from the start of the P wave to the start of the QRS complex. This represents the inbuilt delay in electrical conduction at the atrioventricular (AV) node. Normally <0.20 seconds (5 small squares at standard recording speed).
- QRS complex: the width of the QRS complex. Normally <0.12 seconds (3 small squares at standard rate).
- R–R interval: from the peak of one R wave to the next. This is used in the calculation of heart rate.
- QT interval: from the start of the QRS complex to the end of the T wave. Varies with heart rate. Corrected QT = QT/square root of the R–R interval. Corrected QT interval should be 0.38–0.42 seconds.

Rhythm

- Is the rhythm (and the time between successive R waves) regular or irregular?
  - If irregular but in a clear pattern, then it is said to be 'regularly irregular' (e.g. types of heart block)
  - If irregular but no pattern, then it is said to be 'irregularly irregular' (e.g. atrial fibrillation).

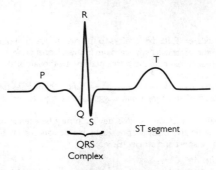

Fig. 5.5 The basic shape of a typical ECG trace.

ECG axis

Cardiac axis

The cardiac axis, or 'QRS axis', refers to the overall direction of depolarization through the ventricular myocardium in the coronal plane.

Zero degrees is taken as the horizontal line to the left of the heart (the right of your diagram).

The normal cardiac axis lies between −30 and +90 degrees (see Fig. 5.6). An axis outside of this range may suggest pathology, either congenital or acquired.

Note, however, that cardiac axis deviation may be seen in healthy individuals with distinctive body shapes. Right axis deviation if tall and thin; left axis deviation if short and stocky (Box 5.1).

Calculating the axis

Look at Fig. 5.7. Leads I, II, and III all lie in the coronal plane (along with aVR, aVL, and aVF). By calculating the relative depolarization in each of these directions, one can calculate the cardiac axis. To accurately determine the cardiac axis, you should use leads I, II, and III as described in Fig. 5.7. There are less reliable short cuts, however.

* Draw a diagram like Fig. 5.6 showing the 3 leads—be careful to use the correct angles.
* Look at the ECG lead I. Count the number of mm above the baseline that the QRS complex reaches.
* Subtract from this the number of mm below the baseline that the QRS complex reaches.
* Now measure this number of centimetres along line I on your diagram and make a mark (measure backward for negative numbers).
* Repeat this for leads II and III.
* Extend lines from your marks, perpendicular to the leads (see Fig. 5.6).
* The direction from the centre of the diagram to the point at which all these lines meet is the cardiac axis.

Calculating the axis—short cuts

There are many shorter ways of roughly calculating the cardiac axis. These are less accurate, however.

An easy method is to look at only leads I and aVF. These are perpendicular to each other and make a simpler diagram than the one described above.

An even easier method is to look at the print-out. Most computerized machines will now tell you the ECG axis (but you should still have an understanding of the theory behind it).

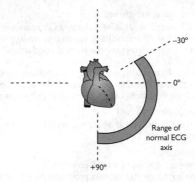

Fig. 5.6 The normal ECG axis.

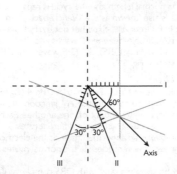

Fig. 5.7 Calculating the ECG axis using leads I, II, and III. See text.

Box 5.1 Some causes of axis deviation

Left axis deviation (<–30 degrees)

- Left ventricular hypertrophy
- Left bundle branch block (LBBB)
- Left anterior hemiblock (anterior fascicle of the left bundle)
- Inferior myocardial infarction
- Cardiomyopathies
- Tricuspid atresia.

Right axis deviation (>+90 degrees)

- Right ventricular hypertrophy
- Right bundle branch block (RBBB)
- Anterolateral myocardial infarction
- Right ventricular strain (e.g. pulmonary embolism)
- Cor pulmonale
- Fallot's tetralogy (pulmonary stenosis).

AV conduction abnormalities

In the normal ECG each P wave is followed by a QRS complex. The isoelectric gap between is the PR interval and represents slowing of the impulse at the AV junction. Disturbance of the normal conduction here, leads to 'heart block' (Fig. 5.8).

Causes of heart block include ischaemic heart disease, idiopathic fibrosis of the conduction system, cardiomyopathies, inferior and anterior MI, drugs (digoxin, β-blockers, verapamil), and physiological (1st degree) in athletes.

First degree heart block

PR interval fixed but prolonged at >0.20 seconds (5 small squares at standard rate). See rhythm strip 1 (Fig. 5.8).

Second degree heart block

Not every P wave is followed by a QRS complex.

- Möbitz type I: PR interval becomes progressively longer after each P wave until an impulse fails to be conducted at all. The interval then returns to the normal length and the cycle is repeated (rhythm strip 2, Fig. 5.8). This is also known as the Wenckebach phenomenon.
- Möbitz type II: PR interval is fixed but not every P wave is followed by a QRS. The relationship between P waves and QRS complex may be 2:1 (2 P waves for every QRS), 3:1 (3 P waves per QRS), or random. See rhythm strip 3, Fig. 5.8.

Third degree heart block

Also called complete heart block. See rhythm strip 4 (Fig. 5.8). There is no conduction of the impulse through the AV junction. Atrial and ventricular depolarization occur independent of one another. Each has a separate pacemaker triggering electrical activity at different rates.

- The QRS complex is an abnormal shape as the electrical impulse does not travel through the ventricles via the normal routes (see ventricular escape).
- P waves may be seen 'merging' with QRS complexes if they coincide.

Notes

- If in doubt about the pattern of P waves and QRS complexes, mark out the P wave intervals and the R–R intervals separately, then compare.
- P waves are best seen in leads II and V_1.

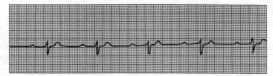

Rhythm strip 1—first degree heart block.

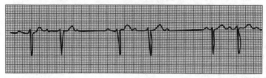

Rhythm strip 2—second degree heart block Möbitz type I.

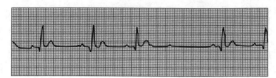

Rhythm strip 3—second degree heart block Möbitz type II.

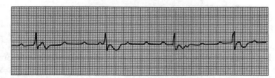

Rhythm strip 4—third degree (complete) heart block.

Fig. 5.8 Rhythm strips showing AV conduction abnormalities.

Ventricular conduction abnormalities

Depolarization of both ventricles usually occurs rapidly through left and right bundle branches of the His–Purkinje system (see Fig. 5.9). If this process is disrupted as a result of damage to the conducting system, depolarization will occur more slowly through non-specialized ventricular myocardium. The QRS complex—usually <0.12 seconds' duration—will become prolonged and is described as a 'broad' (Fig. 5.9).

Right bundle branch block (RBBB)

Conduction through the AV node, bundle of His, and left bundle branch will be normal but depolarization of the right ventricle occurs by the slow spread of electrical current through myocardial cells. The result is delayed right ventricular depolarization giving a second R wave known as R' ('R prime').

RBBB suggests pathology in the right side of the heart but can be a normal variant (Fig. 5.10).

ECG changes

(See Box 5.2 for bundle branch block mnemonic.)

- 'RSR' pattern seen in V_1.
- Cardiac axis usually remains normal unless left anterior fascicle is also blocked ('bifascicular block') which results in left axis deviation.
- T wave flattening or inversion in anterior chest leads (V_1–V_3).

Some causes of RBBB

- Hyperkalaemia.
- Congenital heart disease (e.g. Fallot's tetralogy).
- Pulmonary embolus.
- Cor pulmonale.
- Fibrosis of conduction system.

Left bundle branch block (LBBB)

Conduction through the AV node, bundle of His, and right bundle branch will be normal but depolarization of the left ventricle occurs by the slow spread of electrical current through myocardial cells. The result is delayed left ventricular depolarization (Fig. 5.11).

LBBB should always be considered pathological.

ECG changes

- 'M' pattern seen in V_6.
- T wave flattening or inversion in lateral chest leads (V_5–V_6).

Some causes of LBBB

- Hypertension.
- Ischaemic heart disease.
- Acute myocardial infarction.
- Aortic stenosis.
- Cardiomyopathies.
- Fibrosis of conduction system.

🛈 LBBB on the ECG causes abnormalities of the ST segment and T wave. You should not comment any further on these parts of the trace.

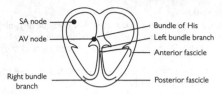

Fig. 5.9 Diagrammatic representation of the conducting system of the heart.

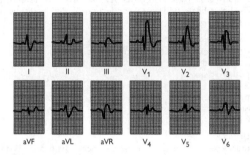

Fig. 5.10 Typical 12-lead ECG showing RBBB.

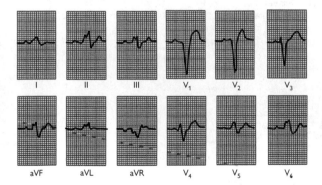

Fig. 5.11 Typical 12-lead ECG showing LBBB.

Box 5.2 Bundle branch block mnemonic

- LBBB, the QRS complex in V_1 looks like a 'W' and an 'M' in V_6. This can be remembered as 'WiLLiaM'. There is a W at the start, an M at the end and 'L' in the middle for 'left'
- Conversely, in the case of RBBB, the QRS complex in V_1 looks like an 'M' and a 'W' in V_6. Combined with an 'R' for right, you have the word 'MaRRoW'.

Sinus rhythms

Supraventricular rhythms arise in the atria. They may be physiological in the case of some causes of sinus brady- and tachycardia or may be caused by pathology within the SA node, the atria, or the first parts of the conducting system.

Normal conduction through the bundle of His into the ventricles will usually give narrow QRS complexes.

Sinus bradycardia

This is a bradycardia (rate <60 beats per minute) at the level of the SA node. The heart beats slowly but conduction of the impulse is normal. (Rhythm strip 1, Fig. 5.12.)

Some causes of sinus bradycardia

- Drugs (β-blockers, verapamil, amiodarone, digoxin).
- Sick sinus syndrome.
- Hypothyroidism.
- Inferior MI.
- Hypothermia.
- Raised intracranial pressure.
- Physiological (athletes).

Sinus tachycardia

This is a tachycardia at the level of the SA node—the heart is beating too quickly but conduction of the impulse is normal. (Rhythm strip 2, Fig. 5.12.)

ECG features

- Ventricular rate > 100 (usually 100–150 beats per minute).
- Normal P wave before each QRS.

Some causes of sinus tachycardia

- Drugs (epinephrine/adrenaline, caffeine, nicotine).
- Pain.
- Exertion.
- Anxiety.
- Anaemia.
- Thyrotoxicosis.
- Pulmonary embolus.
- Hepatic failure.
- Cardiac failure.
- Hypercapnia.
- Pregnancy.
- Constrictive pericarditis.

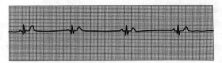

Rhythm strip 1—sinus bradycardia.

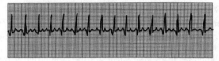

Rhythm strip 2—sinus tachycardia.

Fig. 5.12 Rhythm strips from lead II showing a sinus bradycardia (rhythm strip 1) and sinus tachycardia (rhythm strip 2).

Supraventricular tachycardias

These are tachycardias (rate >100bpm) arising in the atria or the AV node. As conduction through the bundle of His and ventricles will be normal (unless there is other pathology in the heart), the QRS complexes appear normal (Fig. 5.13).

There are four main causes of a supraventricular tachycardia that you should be aware of: atrial fibrillation, atrial flutter, junctional tachycardia, and re-entry tachycardia.

Atrial fibrillation (AF)

This is disorganized contraction of the atria in the form of rapid, irregular twitching. There will, therefore, be no P waves on the ECG.

Electrical impulses from the twitches of the atria arrive at the AV node randomly, they are then conducted via the normal pathways to cause ventricular contraction. The result is a characteristic ventricular rhythm that is *irregularly irregular* with no discernible pattern.

ECG features

- No P waves. Rhythm is described as *irregularly irregular*.
- Irregular QRS complexes.
- Normal appearance of QRS.
- Ventricular rate may be increased ('fast AF')—typically 120–160 per minute.

Some causes of atrial fibrillation

- Idiopathic.
- Ischaemic heart disease.
- Thyroid disease.
- Hypertension.
- MI.
- Pulmonary embolus.
- Rheumatic mitral or tricuspid valve disease.

Atrial flutter

This is the abnormally rapid contraction of the atria. The contractions are not disorganized or random, unlike AF, but are fast and inadequate for the normal movement of blood. Instead of P waves, the baseline will have a typical 'saw-tooth' appearance (sometimes known as F waves).

The AV node is unable to conduct impulses faster than 200/min. Atrial contraction faster than that leads to impulses failing to be conducted. For example, an atrial rate of 300/min will lead to every other impulse being conducted giving a ventricular rate (and pulse) of 150/min. In this case, it is called '2:1 block'. Other ratios of atrial to ventricular contractions may occur.

A variable block at the AV node may lead to an irregularly irregular pulse indistinguishable from that of AF on clinical examination.

ECG features

- 'Saw-tooth' appearance of baseline.
- Normal appearance of QRS complexes.

Causes of atrial flutter

- Similar to AF.

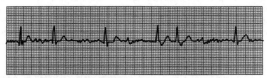

Rhythm strip 1—atrial fibrillation.

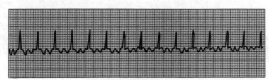

Rhythm strip 2—atrial flutter with 2:1 block.

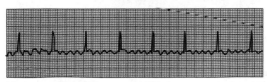

Rhythm strip 3—atrial flutter with 4:1 block.

Fig. 5.13 Rhythm strips from lead II showing some supraventricular tachycardias.

Junctional (nodal) tachycardia

The area in or around the AV node depolarizes spontaneously, the impulse will be immediately conducted to the ventricles. The QRS complex will be of a normal shape but no P waves will be seen.

ECG features

- No P waves.
- QRS complexes are regular and normal shape.
- Rate may be fast or may be of a normal rate.

Some causes of junctional tachycardia

- Sick sinus syndrome (including drug-induced).
- Digoxin toxicity.
- Ischaemia of the AV node, especially with acute inferior MI.
- Acutely after cardiac surgery.
- Acute inflammatory processes (e.g. acute rheumatic fever) which may involve the conduction system.
- Diphtheria.
- Other drugs (e.g. most anti-arrhythmic agents).

Wolff–Parkinson–White syndrome

In Wolff–Parkinson–White (WPW) syndrome, there is an extra conducting pathway between the atria and the ventricles (the bundle of Kent)—a break in the normal electrical insulation. This 'accessory' pathway is not specialized for conducting electrical impulses so does not delay the impulse as the AV node does. However, it is not linked to the normal conduction pathways of the bundle of His.

Depolarization of the ventricles will occur partly via the AV node and partly by the bundle of Kent. During normal atrial contraction, electrical activity reaches the AV node and the accessory pathway at roughly the same time. Whilst it is held up temporarily at the AV node, the impulse passes through the accessory pathway and starts to depolarize the ventricles via non-specialized cells ('pre-excitation'), distorting the first part of the R wave and giving a short PR interval. Normal conduction via the bundle of His then supervenes. The result is a slurred upstroke of the QRS complex called a 'delta wave'.

This is an example of a 'fusion beat' in which normal and abnormal ventricular depolarization combine to give a distortion of the QRS complex (Fig. 5.14 and Box 5.3).

Re-entry tachycardia

The accessory pathway may allow electrical activity to be conducted from the ventricles back up to the atria.

For example, in a re-entry tachycardia, electrical activity may be conducted down the bundle of His, across the ventricles and up the accessory pathway into the atria causing them to contract again, and the cycle is repeated. This is called a 're-entry circuit' (Figs 5.15 and 5.16).

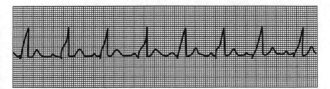

Fig. 5.14 Rhythm strip showing Wolff–Parkinson–White syndrome.

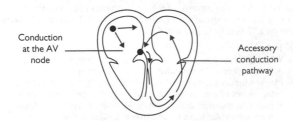

Conduction at the AV node

Accessory conduction pathway

Fig. 5.15 Diagrammatic representation of re-entry tachycardia.

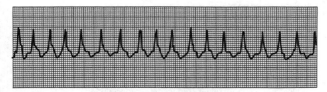

Fig. 5.16 Rhythm strip showing a re-entry tachycardia.

Box 5.3 Classification of Wolff–Parkinson–White syndrome

The bundle of Kent may connect the atria with either the right or the left ventricle. Thus, WPW is classically divided into two groups according to the resulting appearance of the QRS complex in the anterior chest leads. In practice, this classification is rather simplistic as 11% of patients may have more than one accessory pathway.

- *Type A:* upright delta wave and QRS in V_1
  - May be mistaken for RBBB or posterior MI.
- *Type B:* downward delta wave and QRS in V_1, positive elsewhere.

Ventricular rhythms

Most ventricular rhythms originate outside the usual conduction pathways meaning that excitation spreads by an abnormal path through the ventricular muscle to give broad or unusually shaped QRS complexes (Fig. 5.17).

Ventricular tachycardia (VT)

Here, there is a focus of ventricular tissue depolarizing rapidly within the ventricular myocardium. VT is defined as 3 or more successive ventricular extrasystoles at a rate of >120/min. 'Sustained' VTs last for >30 secs.

VT may be 'stable' showing a repetitive QRS shape ('monomorphic') or unstable with varying patterns of the QRS complex ('polymorphic').

It may be impossible to distinguish VT from an SVT with bundle branch block on a 12-lead ECG (see also Box 5.5).

ECG features

- Wide QRS complexes which are irregular in rhythm and shape.
- A-V dissociation—independent atrial and ventricular contraction.
- May see fusion and capture beats on ECG as signs of atrial activity independent of the ventricular activity—said to be pathognomonic.
  - Fusion beats: depolarization from AV node meets depolarization from ventricular focus causing hybrid QRS complex.
  - Capture beats: atrial beat conducted to ventricles causing a normal QRS complex in amongst the VT trace.
- Rate can be up to 130–300/min.
- QRS concordance: all the QRS complexes in the chest leads are either mainly positive or mainly negative—this suggests a ventricular origin of the tachycardia.
- Extreme axis deviation (far negative or far positive).

Some causes of ventricular tachycardia

- Ischaemia (acute including MI or chronic).
- Electrolyte abnormalities (reduced K^+, reduced Mg^{2+}).
- Aggressive adrenergic stimulation (e.g. cocaine use).
- Drugs—especially anti-arrhythmics.

Ventricular fibrillation (VF)

This is disorganized, uncoordinated depolarization from multiple foci in the ventricular myocardium (Box 5.4).

ECG features

- No discernible QRS complexes.
- A completely disorganized ECG.

Some causes of ventricular fibrillation

- Coronary heart disease.
- Cardiac inflammatory diseases.
- Abnormal metabolic states.
- Pro-arrhythmic toxic exposures.
- Electrocution.
- Tension pneumothorax, trauma, and drowning.
- Large pulmonary embolism.
- Hypoxia or acidosis.

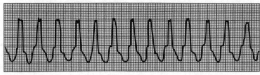

Rhythm strip 1—monomorphic ventricular tachycardia (VT).

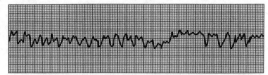

Rhythm strip 2—ventricular fibrillation (VF).

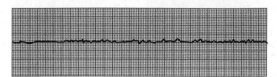

Rhythm strip 3—'fine' ventricular fibrillation.

Fig. 5.17 Rhythm strips showing ventricular rhythms.

Box 5.4 Fine VF

This is VF with a small amplitude waveform. It may resemble asystole on the ECG monitor (see Fig. 5.19), particularly in an emergency situation.

In a clinical situation, you should remember to increase the gain on the monitor to ensure what you think is asystole is not really fine VF as the management for each is very different.

Other ventricular rhythms

Ventricular extrasystoles (ectopics)

These are ventricular contractions originating from a focus of depolarization within the ventricle. As conduction is via abnormal pathways, the QRS complex will be unusually shaped (Fig. 5.19).

Ventricular extrasystoles are common and harmless if there is no structural heart disease. If they occur at the same time as a T wave, the 'R-on-T' phenomenon, they can lead to VF.

Ventricular escape rhythm

This occurs as a 'back-up' when conduction between the atria and the ventricles is interrupted (as in complete heart block).

The intrinsic pacemaker in ventricular myocardium depolarizes at a slow rate (30–40/min).

The ventricular beats will be abnormal and wide with abnormal T waves following them. This rhythm can be stable but may suddenly fail.

Asystole

This is a complete absence of electrical activity and is not compatible with life.

There may be a slight wavering of the baseline which can be easily confused with fine VF in emergency situations.

Agonal rhythm

This is a slow, irregular rhythm with wide ventricular complexes which vary in shape. This is often seen in the later stages of unsuccessful resuscitation attempts as the heart dies. The complexes become progressively broader before all recognizable activity is lost (asystole).

Box 5.5 Torsades de pointes

Torsades de pointes, literally meaning 'twisting of points', is a form of polymorphic VT characterized by a gradual change in the amplitude and twisting of the QRS axis. In the US, it is known as 'cardiac ballet'.

Torsades usually terminates spontaneously but frequently recurs and may degenerate into sustained VT and ventricular fibrillation (Fig. 5.18).

Torsades results from a prolonged QT interval. Causes include congenital long-QT syndromes and drugs (e.g. anti-arrhythmics). Patients may also have reduced K^+ and Mg^{2+}.

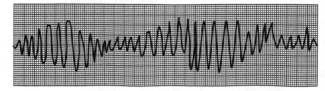

Fig. 5.18 Rhythm strip showing torsades.

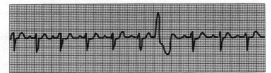

Rhythm strip 1—a single ventricular extrasystole.

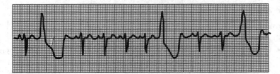

Rhythm strip 2—multiple, unifocal, ventricular extrasystole.

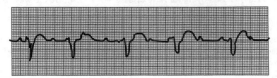

Rhythm strip 3—ventricular escape in the case of complete heart block.

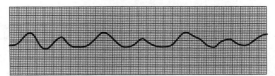

Rhythm strip 4—agonal rhythm.

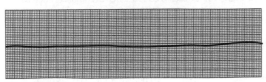

Rhythm strip 5—asystole.

Fig. 5.19 Rhythm strips showing ventricular rhythms.

P and T wave abnormalities

The P wave

Represents depolarization of the small muscle mass of the atria. The P wave is thus much smaller in amplitude than the QRS complex.

Normal

- In sinus rhythm each P wave is closely associated with a QRS complex.
- P waves are usually upright in most leads except aVR.
- P waves are <3 small squares wide and <3 small squares high.

Abnormal

- Right atrial hypertrophy will cause tall, peaked P waves.
  - Causes include pulmonary hypertension (in which case the wave is known as 'P pulmonale') and tricuspid valve stenosis.
- Left atrial hypertrophy will cause the P wave to become wider and twin-peaked or 'bifid'.
  - Usually caused by mitral valve disease—in which case the wave is known as 'P mitrale'.

The T wave

Represents repolarization of the ventricles. The T wave is most commonly affected by ischaemic changes. The most common abnormality is 'inversion' which has a number of causes.

Normal

- Commonly inverted in V_1 and aVR.
- May be inverted in V_1–V_3 as normal variant.

Abnormal

- Myocardial ischaemia or MI (e.g. non-Q wave MI) can cause T wave inversion. Changes need to be interpreted in light of clinical picture (Fig. 5.20).
- Ventricular hypertrophy causes T inversion in those leads focused on the ventricle in question. For example, left ventricular hypertrophy will give T changes in leads V_5, V_6, II, and aVL.
- Bundle branch block causes abnormal QRS complexes due to abnormal pathways of ventricular depolarization. The corresponding abnormal repolarization gives unusually shaped T waves which have no significance in themselves.
- Digoxin causes a characteristic T wave inversion with a downsloping of the ST segment known as the 'reverse tick' sign. This occurs at therapeutic doses and is not a sign of digoxin toxicity.
- Electrolyte imbalances cause a number of T wave changes:
  - Raised K^+ can cause tall tented T waves
  - Low K^+ can cause small T waves and U waves (broad, flat waves occurring after the T waves)
  - Low Ca^{2+} can cause small T waves with a prolongation of the QT interval. (Raised Ca^{2+} has the reverse effect)
  - Other causes of T wave inversion include subarachnoid haemorrhage and lithium use.

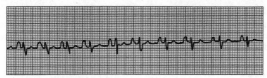

Rhythm strip 1—peaked P waves.

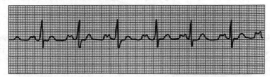

Rhythm strip 2—bifid P waves.

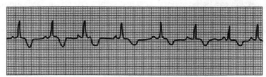

Rhythm strip 3—T wave inversion after myocardial infarction.

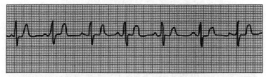

Rhythm strip 4—hyperkalaemia with peaked T waves.

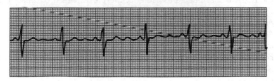

Rhythm strip 5—hyperkalaemia with small T waves and U waves.

Fig. 5.20 Rhythm strips showing some P and T wave abnormalities.

The ST segment

This is the portion of the ECG from the end of the QRS complex to the start of the T wave and is an isoelectric line in the normal ECG. Changes in the ST segment can represent myocardial ischaemia and, most importantly, acute MI (Fig. 5.21).

ST elevation

The degree and extent of ST elevation is of crucial importance in ECG interpretation as it determines whether reperfusion therapy (thrombolysis or primary PCI) is considered in acute MI.

Causes of ST elevation

- Acute MI—convex ST elevation in affected leads (the 'tomb-stone' appearance), often with reciprocal ST depression in opposite leads.
- Pericarditis—widespread concave ST elevation ('saddle-shaped').
- Left ventricular aneurysm—ST elevation may persist over time.

ST depression

ST depression can be horizontal, upward sloping, or downward sloping.

Causes of ST depression

- Myocardial ischaemia—horizontal ST depression and an upright T wave. May be result of coronary artery disease or other causes (e.g. anaemia, aortic stenosis).
- Digoxin toxicity—downward sloping ('reverse tick').
- 'Non-specific' changes—ST segment depression which is often upward sloping may be a normal variant and is not thought to be associated with any underlying significant pathology.

Myocardial infarction

In the first hour following a MI, the ECG can remain normal. However, when changes occur, they usually develop in the following order:
- ST segment becomes elevated and T waves become peaked.
- Pathological Q waves develop.
- ST segment returns to baseline and T waves invert.

The leads in which these changes take place allow you to identify which part of the heart has been affected and, therefore, which coronary artery is likely to be occluded.
- *Anterior:* V_2–V_5.
- *Antero-lateral:* I, aVL, V_5, V_6.
- *Inferior:* III, aVF (sometimes II also).
- *Posterior:* the usual depolarization of the posterior of the left ventricle is lost, giving a dominant R wave in V_1. Imagine it as a mirror image of the Q wave you would expect with an anterior infarction.
- *Right ventricular:* often no changes on the 12-lead ECG. If suspected clinically, leads are placed on the right of the chest, mirroring the normal pattern and are labelled V_1R, V_2R, V_3R, and so on.

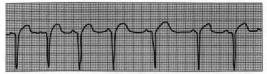

Rhythm strip 1—lead V$_2$ showing acute myocardial infarction.

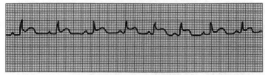

Rhythm strip 2—pericarditis. The ST elevation is usually described as 'saddle-shaped'.

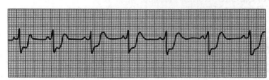

Rhythm strip 3—ischaemia.

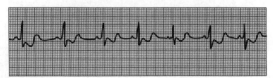

Rhythm strip 4—digoxin use showing the 'reverse tick'.

Fig. 5.21 Rhythm strips showing some ST segment abnormalities.

Hypertrophy

If the heart is faced with having to overcome pressure overload (e.g. left ventricular hypertrophy in hypertension or aortic stenosis) or higher systemic pressures (e.g. essential hypertension) then it will increase its muscle mass in response. This increased muscle mass can result in changes to the ECG.

Atrial hypertrophy

This can lead to changes to the P wave.

Ventricular hypertrophy

This can lead to changes to the cardiac axis, QRS complex height/depth, and the T wave.

Left ventricular hypertrophy (LVH)

- Tall R wave in V_6 and deep S wave in V_1.
- May also see left axis deviation.
- T wave inversion in V_5, V_6, I, aVL.
- Voltage criteria for LVH include:
  - R wave >25mm (5 large squares) in V_6
  - R wave in V_6 + S wave in V_1 >35mm (7 large squares).

Right ventricular hypertrophy

- 'Dominant' R wave in V_1 (i.e. R wave bigger than S wave).
- Deep S wave in V_6.
- May also see right axis deviation.
- T wave inversion in V_1–V_3.

Paced rhythms

Temporary or permanent cardiac pacing may be indicated for a number of conditions such as complete heart block or symptomatic bradycardia. These devices deliver a tiny electrical pulse to an area of the heart, initiating contraction. This can be seen on the ECG as a sharp spike (Fig. 5.22).

Many different types of pacemaker exist, and can be categorized according to:

- The chamber paced (atria or ventricles or both).
- The chamber used to detect the heart's electrical activity (atria or ventricles or both).
- How the pacemaker responds—most are inhibited by the normal electrical activity of the heart.

On the ECG look for the pacing spikes which may appear before P waves if the atria are paced, before the QRS complexes if the ventricles are paced, or both.

🛈 Be careful not to mistake the vertical lines that separate the different leads on some ECG print-outs as pacing spikes!

▶ Paced complexes do not show the expected changes described elsewhere in this section. You are, therefore, unable to diagnose ischaemia in the presence of pacing.

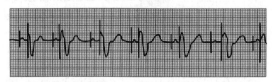

Fig. 5.22 Rhythm strip showing dual chamber pacing.

Peak expiratory flow rate (PEFR)

Peak expiratory flow rate (PEFR) is the maximum flow rate recorded during a forced expiration. Predicted readings vary depending on age, sex, height, and ethnicity (Fig. 5.23).

See ➔ Chapter 4 for how to perform this test.
See Boxes 5.6 and 5.7 for other tests.

Interpreting PEFR

PEFR readings less than the patient's predicted, or usual best, demonstrate airflow obstruction in the large airways.

PEFR readings are useful in determining the severity, and therefore the most appropriate treatment algorithm, for asthma exacerbations:

- PEFR <75% best or predicted—moderate asthma attack.
- PEFR <50% best or predicted—acute severe asthma attack.
- PEFR <33% best or predicted—life-threatening asthma attack.

Reversibility testing

Improvement in PEFR or FEV_1 ≥15% following bronchodilator therapy (e.g. salbutamol) shows reversibility of airflow obstruction and can help to distinguish asthma from poorly reversible conditions such as COPD.

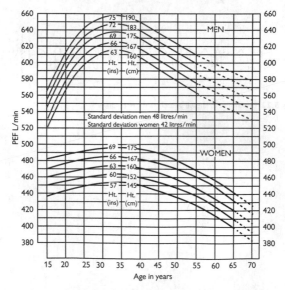

Fig. 5.23 Normal PEFR by age and gender. Image reproduced from the *Oxford Handbook of Clinical Medicine*, with permission.

Box 5.6 Gas transfer

- This test measures the capacity of a gas to diffuse across the alveolar–capillary membranes. This not only adds further clues to the nature of the lung disease but is also a measure of function which can give important prognostic information and help guide treatment
- DLCO (carbon monoxide diffusion capacity) measures the uptake from a single breath of 0.3% CO
- DLCO is reduced in interstitial lung disease (the fibrotic insterstitium limits gas diffusion) and emphysema (the total surface area available for gas transfer is reduced).

Box 5.7 Other lung function tests

Specialized lung function centres can calculate static lung volumes with a body plethysmograph or using helium rebreathe and dilutional techniques including:

- TLC—total lung capacity
- RV— residual volume.

Both can help when identifying patterns of lung disease and help assess patients prior to lung surgery.

Basic spirometry

Spirometry measures airflow and functional lung volumes; this can aid diagnosis of a number of conditions, but is primarily used to distinguish between restrictive and obstructive lung diseases.

Patients are asked to blow, as fast as possible, into a mouthpiece attached to a spirometer. This records the rate and volume of airflow.

Most spirometers are now hand-held computerized devices which will print a spirometry report for you and calculate normal values.

Two key values are:
- FEV_1: forced expiratory volume in the first second.
- FVC: forced vital capacity—the total lung volume from maximum inspiration to maximum expiration, in forced exhalation.

Flow volume loops can also be generated from spirometry data and show the flow at different lung volumes. These are useful in distinguishing intra- and extra-thoracic causes of obstruction as well as to assess for small air-ways obstruction (Figs 5.24 and 5.25).

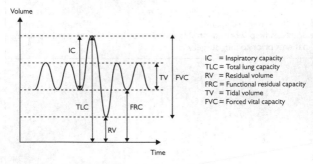

IC = Inspiratory capacity
TLC = Total lung capacity
RV = Residual volume
FRC = Functional residual capacity
TV = Tidal volume
FVC = Forced vital capacity

Fig. 5.24 Normal pattern of lung volumes.

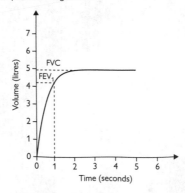

Fig. 5.25 Spirogram showing normal volume–time graph.

Common patterns of abnormality

Obstructive

When airflow is obstructed, although FVC may be reduced, FEV_1 is much more reduced, hence the FEV_1/FVC ratio falls. It can also take much longer to fully exhale. Note that FVC can be normal in mild/moderate obstructive conditions.

Conditions causing an obstructive defect include COPD, asthma, and bronchiectasis as well as foreign bodies, tumours, and stenosis following tracheotomy (all localized airflow obstruction).

Restrictive

The airway patency is not affected in restrictive lung conditions, so the PEFR can be normal. But the FEV_1 and FVC are reduced due to the restrictive picture.

Conditions causing a restrictive defect include fibrosing alveolitis of any cause, skeletal abnormalities (e.g. kyphoscoliosis), neuromuscular diseases (e.g. motor neuron disease), connective tissue diseases, late-stage sarcoidosis, pleural effusion, and pleural thickening (Table 5.1 and Fig. 5.26).

Table 5.1 Obstructive vs restrictive spirometry results

Pattern	FEV_1	FVC	FEV_1/FVC ratio	TLC	RV
Obstructive	↓	↔/↓	<75%	↑ (or ↔)	↑
Restrictive	↓	↓	>75%	↓	↓

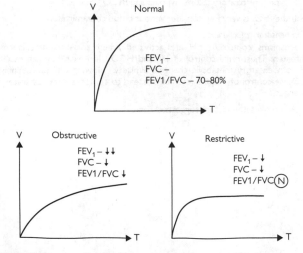

Fig. 5.26 Spirograms showing obstructive and restrictive volume/time curves.

Arterial blood gas analysis

A systematic approach

The printout from the ABG machine can have a bewildering number of results. Initially, just focus on the pH, $PaCO_2$, and HCO_3^- in that order (Box 5.8):

pH
- Is it low (acidosis) or high (alkalosis)?

$PaCO_2$
- If $PaCO_2$ is raised and there is acidosis (pH <7.35) you can deduce a respiratory acidosis.
- If $PaCO_2$ is low and there is alkalosis (pH >7.45) then the lack of acid gas has led to a respiratory alkalosis.
- If $PaCO_2$ is low and there is acidosis then the respiratory system will not be to blame and there is a metabolic acidosis.
  - Confirm this by looking at the HCO_3^-, it should be low.
- If $PaCO_2$ is high or normal and there is alkalosis, there must be a *metabolic alkalosis*.
  - Confirm this by looking at the HCO_3^-, it should be raised.

PaO_2

❶ Note what FiO_2 the patient was breathing when the sample was taken.

Hypoxia is PaO_2 of <8.0kPa and can result from a ventilation–perfusion mismatch (e.g. pulmonary embolism) or from alveolar hypoventilation (e.g. COPD, pneumonia).
- Type I respiratory failure: hypoxia and $PaCO_2$ <6kPa.
- Type II respiratory failure: hypoxia and $PaCO_2$ >6kPa.

▶ If the PaO_2 is very low consider venous blood contamination.

Compensatory mechanisms

Mechanisms controlling pH are activated when acid–base imbalances threaten. Thus, renal control of H^+ and HCO_3^- ion excretion can result in compensatory metabolic changes. Similarly, 'blowing off' or retaining CO_2 via control of respiratory rate can lead to compensatory respiratory changes.

▶ A compensated picture suggests chronic disease.

Box 5.8 Reference ranges
- pH 7.35–7.45
- $PaCO_2$ 4.7–6.0kPa
- PaO_2 10–13kPa
- HCO_3^- 22–26mmol/L
- Base excess −2 to +2.

Table 5.2 Obstructive vs restrictive spirometry results

Pattern	pH	TLC	RV
Respiratory acidosis	↓	↑	↔ (↑ if compensated)
Metabolic acidosis	↓	↔ (↓ if compensated)	↓
Respiratory alkalosis	↑	↓	↔ (↓ if compensated)
Metabolic alkalosis	↑	↔ (↑ if compensated)	↑

Box 5.9 Anion gap
- $(Na^+ + K^+) − (HCO_3^- + Cl^-)$
- Normal range = 10–18 mmol/L.

Acidosis

A relative excess of cations (e.g. H^+), unless adequately compensated, will result in acidosis (more correctly acidaemia) (Table 5.2).

Respiratory acidosis
- pH ↓.
- $PaCO_2$ ↑.
- HCO_3^- may be ↑ if compensated.

Conditions which can lead to respiratory acidosis:
- COPD, asthma, pneumonia, pneumothorax, pulmonary fibrosis.
- Obstructive sleep apnoea.
- Opiate overdose (causing respiratory depression).
- Neuromuscular disorders (e.g. Guillain–Barré, motor neuron disease).
- Skeletal abnormalities (e.g. kyphoscoliosis).
- Congestive cardiac failure.

Metabolic acidosis
- pH ↓.
- HCO_3^- ↓.
- $PaCO_2$ may be ↓ if compensated.

It is useful to calculate the anion gap to help distinguish causes of metabolic acidosis (Box 5.9).

An increased anion gap points to increased production of immeasurable anions.

Conditions which can lead to metabolic acidosis:
- Raised anion gap.
  - Diabetic ketoacidosis
  - Renal failure (urate)
  - Lactic acidosis (tissue hypoxia or excessive exercise)
  - Salicylates, ethylene glycol, biguanides.
- Normal anion gap.
  - Chronic diarrhoea, ileostomy (loss of HCO_3^-)
  - Addison's disease
  - Pancreatic fistulae
  - Renal tubular acidosis
  - Acetazolamide treatment (loss of HCO_3^-).

Alkalosis

A relative excess of anions (e.g. HCO_3^-), unless adequately compensated, will result in alkalosis (more correctly alkalaemia). (See Box 5.10.)

Respiratory alkalosis

- pH ↑.
- $PaCO_2$ ↓.
- HCO_3^- may be ↓ if compensated.

Conditions which can lead to respiratory alkalosis:

- Hyperventilation, secondary to:
  - Panic attack (anxiety)
  - Pain.
- Meningitis.
- Stroke, subarachnoid haemorrhage.
- High altitude.

Metabolic alkalosis

- pH ↑.
- HCO_3^- ↑.
- $PaCO_2$ may be ↑ if compensated.

Conditions which can lead to metabolic alkalosis:

- Diuretic drugs (via loss of K^+).
- Prolonged vomiting (via acid replacement and release of HCO_3^-).
- Burns.
- Base ingestion.

Box 5.10 Mixed metabolic and respiratory disturbance

- In clinical practice patients can develop a mixed picture where acid–base imbalance is the result of both respiratory and metabolic factors
- For example, in critically ill patients, hypoventilation leads to low PaO_2, and O_2 depleted cells then produce lactic acid.

Cerebrospinal fluid (CSF)

CSF is produced by the choroid plexus lining the cerebral ventricles and helps cushion and support the brain. Samples are usually obtained by lumbar puncture (see Table 5.3).

Normal adult CSF

- Pressure 6–20cm H_2O.
- Red cells nil.
- Lymphocytes ≤5 x 10^6/L.
- Neutrophils nil.
- Protein <450 mg/L.
- Glucose 2.5–4.0mmol/L (2/3 of blood glucose).
- IgG 5–45mg/L.

▶ CSF glucose is abnormal if <50% of blood glucose level.
❶ Premature babies, newborns, children, and adolescents have different normal ranges.

Table 5.3 Characteristics of CSF according to underlying pathology

Pathology	Appearance	Protein	Glucose (CSF:blood ratio)	Cells
Bacterial meningitis	Turbid	↑	↓	Neutrophils
Viral meningitis	Clear	↔/↑	↑/↔	Lymphocytes
Viral encephalitis	Clear	↔/↑	↓	Lymphocytes
TB meningitis	Fibrin webs		↓↓	Lymphocytes Neutrophils
Fungal meningitis	Clear/turbid		↓	Lymphocytes
Subarachnoid haemorrhage	Xanthochromia	↔/↑	↑	Red cells
Multiple sclerosis	Clear	↔/↑	↔/↑	Lymphocytes
Guillain–Barré syndrome	Clear	↑	↔/↑	
Cord compression	Clear	↑	↔	
Malignancy	Clear	↑	↓	Malignant

Urinalysis

Bedside dipstick urinalysis offers speedy and non-invasive testing that can help with the diagnosis of common conditions such as UTIs and diabetes mellitus. Samples can be sent to the laboratory for further analysis, including MCS.

Dipstick

Dipstick testing gives semi-quantitative analysis of:
- Protein (normally negative).
- Glucose (normally negative).
- Ketones (normally negative).
- Nitrites (normally negative).
- Blood (normally negative).
- Leukocytes (normally negative).
- Bilirubin (normally negative).
- pH (normally acidic with range 4.5–8.0).
- Specific gravity (normal range 1.000–1.030).

Notes on dipstick testing
- ▶ Test the urine within 15 minutes of obtaining the sample.
- ▶ Urine pregnancy testing is equally convenient and is indicated in females of child-bearing age who present with abdominal symptoms.
- ▶ Various foods (e.g. beetroot) and drugs (e.g. rifampicin, tetracyclines, levodopa, phenytoin, chloroquine, iron supplements) can change the colour of urine.

Microscopy, culture, and sensitivity (MCS)

Microscopy allows identification of bacteria and other microorganisms, urinary casts (formed in the tubules or collecting ducts from proteins or cells), crystals, and cells (including renal tubular, transitional epithelial, leukocytes, and red blood cells). Organism growth and antibiotic sensitivities and can also be determined.

▶ Asymptomatic bacteriuria is more common in pregnancy (up to 7%) and can lead to pyelonephritis and potential fetal complications.

Characteristic urinalysis findings
- UTIs: nitrites, leukocytes.
- Diabetes mellitus: glucose.
- Diabetic ketoacidosis: ketones.
- Cholestasis (obstructive jaundice): bilirubin.
- Pre-hepatic jaundice: urobilinogen.
- Glomerulonephritis: protein, blood.
- Renal stones: blood.
- Renal carcinoma: blood.
- Nephrotic syndrome: protein ++.
- Renal TB: leukocytes, no organisms grown (sterile pyuria).
- Sexually transmitted diseases (chlamydia, gonorrhoea): sterile pyuria.

Pleural fluid

Fluid in the pleural space can be classified as:
- Exudate (protein content >30g/L).
- Transudate (protein content <30g/L).

At borderline levels, if the pleural protein is >50% serum protein then the effusion is an exudate. Blood, pus, and chyle (lymph with fat) can also form an effusion. See ➲ Chapter 4.

See Box 5.11 for other tests.

Transudate causes

Transudates are largely cause by increased venous or reduced oncotic pressure.
- Heart failure.
- Hypoproteinaemia (liver failure, malabsorption, nephrotic syndrome).
- Hypothyroidism.
- Constrictive pericarditis.
- Meig's syndrome (ovarian fibroma and pleural effusion).

Exudate causes

Exudates are largely caused by increased capillary permeability.
- Pneumonia.
- Empyema.
- Malignancy (lung, pleura, lymph).
- Pulmonary infarction.
- TB.
- Systemic lupus erythematosus (SLE).
- Rheumatoid arthritis.
- Dressler's syndrome (post MI).

Box 5.11 Other pleural fluid tests
- Microscopy, culture (conventional and TB culture), and sensitivity (Gram stain, Ziehl–Nielsen stain)
- Cytology (malignant cells)
- Biochemistry.
  - Protein
  - Glucose (reduced if rheumatoid or pneumonia related)
  - Amylase (increased in pancreatitis)
  - LDH (lactate dehydrogenase—increased in empyema, malignancy, rheumatoid disease).

Ascitic fluid

Fluid in the peritoneal cavity can result in abdominal distension and breathlessness. As with pleural fluid, analysis of an aspirated sample can aid diagnosis. See ➲ Chapter 4 for ascitic tap guidance. See Box 5.12 for other tests.

Common causes of ascites
- Decompensated liver disease.
- Infection (bacterial peritonitis, TB).
- Malignancy (liver, ovary).
- Right-sided heart failure.
- Pancreatitis.
- Portal vein occlusion.
- Nephrotic syndrome.

Serum/ascites albumin gradient (SAAG)
- SAAG = [serum albumin] − [ascitic fluid albumin].

SAAG >11g/L
- Portal hypertension.
  - Cirrhosis
  - Alcoholic hepatitis
  - Cardiac ascites
  - Budd–Chiari syndrome
  - Portal vein thrombosis
  - Massive liver metastases
  - Acute fatty liver of pregnancy.

SAAG <11g/L
- Infection.
- Malignancy.
- Nephrotic syndrome.
- Pancreatitis.
- Biliary ascites.
- Serositis in connective tissue disease.
- Bowel perforation or infarction.

Box 5.12 Other ascitic fluid tests
- MCS (bacterial peritonitis, TB)
  - Spontaneous bacterial peritonitis = neutrophils >250/mm^3.
- Cytology (malignant cells, macrophages in inflammatory diseases)
- Biochemistry (protein, glucose, amylase).

Further tests you may consider for a patient with ascites include: liver function tests, clotting, urea and electrolytes (U&Es), hepatitis serology, auto-antibodies, ultrasound scan of liver/pelvis, OGD (varices).

Other investigations

Notes

The procedures detailed in this chapter are for information only—to enable the reader to discuss it with their patients, to prepare the patients correctly, and to identify those patients who may or may not be suitable.

▶ The reader is not expected to perform any of these investigations themselves and this chapter is not intended as a resource for those learning how to perform the investigations.

Computed tomography (CT)

Indications
- Indications are manifold and too numerous to list. See 'making best use of a department of clinical radiology' via 🔗 http://www.rcr.ac.uk

Contraindications
- The standard radiation protection precautions apply.
- The patient must be able to lie flat and still.
- Examinations of the chest usually require the patient to hold their breath.

Technology
- The CT scanner (Fig. 6.1) houses an x-ray tube and rows of detectors which spin at 2–3 revolutions per second, creating a force of up to 25g.
- As the patient is moved slowly through the machine, spiral data is acquired which is then converted to 'slices' by the CT software and sent to PACS or a connected workstation for viewing.

Procedure
This depends on the part of the body examined and the indications for the examination.
- If indicated, the patient may be given oral contrast an hour or more before the examination.
- The patient lies (usually supine) on the scanner table.
  - Head-first for head and neck; feet-first for almost everything else.
- 'Scout' views are acquired which are brief swipes across the area of interest. The resultant images are then used by the radiographer to set the parameters for the scan.
- Most examinations involve intravenous iodinated contrast being given. Note that the contrast is not radioactive.
  - This is usually delivered via an intravenous cannula by an automatic pump-injection device, controlled remotely by the radiographer
  - Contrast may be hand-injected immediately before some scans.
- Depending on the part of the body examined, the patient may be asked to hold their breath via speakers in the machine. Microphones within the scanner allow the staff in the control room to hear the patient.
- The scan itself lasts no more than a couple of minutes.
- Time taken to transfer the patient onto the scanner and set up the intravenous injections will vary.

Risks
- Intravenous contrast reactions include anaphylaxis and nephrotoxicity.
  - Intravenous contrast should not be given to patients with renal impairment unless in special circumstances. Check local guidance.
- Extravasation of intravenous contrast (pain, swelling, erythema).

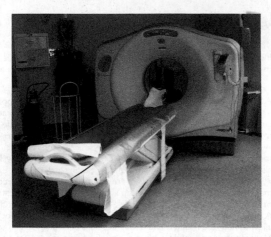

Fig. 6.1 A typical CT scanner. Note the presence of metal in the room (oxygen cylinder, etc.) indicating this is not an MRI scanner and the lead apron indicating that x-rays are being used. The CT scanner has a laser marker (shown) to help with patient positioning, an MRI scanner does not.

Patient preparation
- Fasting: not required for most examinations.

Magnetic resonance imaging (MRI)

Indications
- Indications are manifold and too numerous to list. See 'making best use of a department of clinical radiology' via ℬ http://www.rcr.ac.uk

Contraindications
- As there is no ionizing radiation, radiation precautions do not apply.
- ▶ All ferromagnetic materials will be strongly attracted to the scanner creating missiles which may prove extremely dangerous. MRI-safe trolleys, resuscitation equipment and wheelchairs must be employed.
- ▶ Implanted ferromagnetic devices, aneurysm clips, and retained foreign bodies (e.g. shrapnel or metallic fragments in the eyes) will also move towards the scanner potentially causing major injury.
- ▶ Although electronic pacemakers are not made of ferromagnetic material, they may be 'reset' or stop altogether. The next generation of very new pacemakers is 'MRI safe' – check with the manufacturer.
- A strict questionnaire is employed before anyone (staff or patient) is allowed near the magnet. If in doubt, access is denied.
- Magnetic tape and credit cards may be 'wiped' by the magnet.
- ▶ Many brands of mascara contain ferromagnetic filaments which may heat and cause burns to the eyelids.
- ▶ Caution should also be taken with tattoos; some contain iron.
- The patient must be able to lie flat and still for the duration of the scan.
- Most scanners are relatively tight; larger patients may not fit—check the size and weight limits with your local department.

Technology
- The MRI scanner (Fig. 6.2) houses a very large electromagnet which is always on.
- Radiowaves are produced by the machine which interact with hydrogen atoms in the patient. Radiowaves are, in turn, produced by the interaction with the hydrogen atoms and are detected by the machine which converts the data into images. The scanner has no internal moving parts.

Procedure
- This depends on indications and the part of the body examined.
- The patient lies on the scanner table. 'Coils' may be placed over the body part of interest.
- Most examinations do not involve intravenous contrast being given. If this is given, contrast containing gadolinium (Gd) is usually used.
  - This is usually hand-injected immediately before the scan.
- Depending on the part of the body examined, the patient may be asked to hold their breath via speakers in the machine.
- The scan itself can last up to 40–50 minutes for some body parts.

Risks

- ► *Nephrogenic systemic fibrosis (NSF):* linked to gadolinium exposure in 2006. Symptoms may begin up to 3 months from exposure and may include pain, swelling, erythema, fibrosis of internal organs, and death. Patients with renal impairment are at greatest risk (no cases recorded in those with GFR >60) and at least 9 hours of haemodialysis is required to remove it from the bloodstream. See latest guidance at ℘ http://www.rcr.ac.uk.
- *Metallic artefacts:* twisting or movement of artefacts within the body.
- *Biological effects:* the magnetic fields employed may induce voltages within the body. The most common effect is 'magnetophosphenes' or visual flashes seen by the patient as the optic nerve is stimulated. Stimulation of other nerves and muscles may occur.
- *Tissue burns:* may occur if conducting loops (e.g. ECG leads) are in contact with skin.
- *Temperature:* the oscillating voltages create tissue heating. Overall body temperature may rise by 0.3°C.
- *Noise:* may reach up to 95dB. Headphones or earplugs are usually worn.
- *Claustrophobia:* experienced by up to 10% of patients.

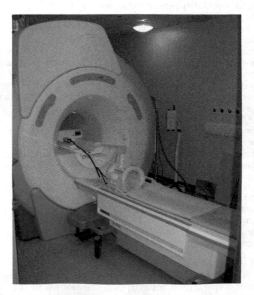

Fig. 6.2 A typical MRI scanner. Note the absence of metal in the room (oxygen cylinder, etc.). A 'coil' is shown within the scanner.

Barium swallow and meal

Barium swallows examine the oropharynx, oesophagus, and gastro-oesophageal junction; barium meals examine the stomach and first part of the duodenum. Swallows and meals are usually performed together as described here.

Indications

- Investigation of oesophageal and gastric pathology. Indications include dysphagia, odynophagia, dyspepsia, weight loss, anaemia, epigastric mass, partial obstruction.
- ▶ Always consider alternatives (e.g. OGD, MRI).

Contraindications

- *Absolute:* lack of informed consent, complete bowel obstruction, suspected perforation (a water-soluble contrast may be used instead).
- *Relative:* a large degree of patient cooperation is required so those unable to understand or follow instructions are unsuitable. Also, the patient must be able to stand for the duration of the examination and to lie supine if necessary.

Procedure

The patient drinks barium whilst the oesophagus and stomach are imaged fluoroscopically. Usually performed by a radiologist.

- The patient stands in the fluoroscopy machine (Fig. 6.3).
- A gas-producing agent is ingested (e.g. Carbex®) and the patient is asked not to belch.
- Images are taken as the patient swallows mouthfuls of barium. The patient must be able to hold the liquid in their mouth and swallow on command.
- Once views of the oesophagus have been obtained, the machine is tilted so the patient is supine. The patient is instructed to roll and tilt as images of the stomach are obtained from several angles.
  - ❶ This requires a certain degree of patient fitness.
- The time taken depends to a degree on how easily the patient follows the commands, although usually lasts 15–20 minutes.
- After the procedure, the patient may eat and drink as usual but is advised to open their bowel regularly to avoid barium impaction.

Risks

- Leakage of barium through an unsuspected perforation.
  - Intraperitoneal and intramediastinal barium has a significant mortality rate.
- Barium impaction (causing large bowel obstruction) or barium appendicitis.

Other information

- ▶ A barium study will prevent a CT examination of the same area for a period of time as intestinal barium creates dense streak artefact.

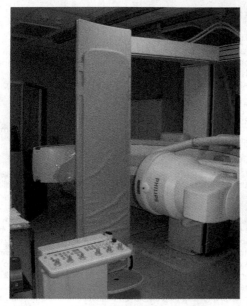

Fig. 6.3 A typical fluoroscopy room set up for an upper gastrointestinal barium examination.

Patient preparation

- *Fasting:* nil by mouth for 6 hours before the examination.
- *Bowel preparation:* none required.
- *Smoking:* patients are asked not to smoke for 6 hours before the procedure as this increases gastric motility.

Water-soluble contrast examinations

- In the case of recent surgery, suspected perforation, or investigation of a leak, water-based iodinated contrast is used instead of barium. Examples include Gastrograffin, Urograffin, Niopam, and Omnipaque.
- A single-contrast examination is performed (i.e. the gas-producing agent is not given) and many of the 'standard' views are not included.
- In contrast to the barium examinations, these studies can be carried out on patients who are frail and/or have recently had surgery.
- Intraperitoneal or intramediastinal water-soluble contrast does not carry the risks of barium but aspiration of the contrast can result in pulmonary oedema and lung fibrosis. Hypersensitivity is also a risk.

Barium follow-through

Indications

- Investigation of small bowel pathology, particularly suspected Crohn's disease and strictures. Indications include pain, diarrhoea, malabsorption, partial obstruction, and anaemia.
- ▶ Always consider alternatives (e.g. MRI, small bowel enema).

Contraindications

- Absolute: lack of informed consent, complete small bowel obstruction, suspected perforation (a water-soluble contrast may be used instead).

Procedure

The patient drinks barium and the small bowel is intermittently imaged until the barium has reached the caecum. Usually performed by a radiologist or senior radiographer.

- The patient is given a mixture of barium to drink.
- The exact mixture given to the patient varies between centres and between radiologists. Some add Gastrograffin to the barium, which has been shown to reduce transit time. Many add 20mg of metoclopramide to the mixture which enhances gastric emptying.
- Once the barium has been consumed, the patient is asked into the fluoroscopy room and images are taken of the small bowel with the patient lying supine (Fig. 6.4).
- Real-time fluoroscopy is employed to assess small bowel motility.
- Images are taken every 20–30 minutes until the barium has reached the colon.
- The radiologist may use a plastic 'spoon' or similar radio-lucent device to press on the patient's abdomen to separate loops of bowel.
- Additional images of the terminal ileum are usually obtained, often with the patient supine, and many radiologists also acquire an 'overcouch' plain abdominal radiograph with compression applied to the lower abdomen.
- The time taken depends on the small bowel transit time and, although usually an hour, patients are advised to allow up to 3 hours for the appointment.
- After the procedure, the patient may eat and drink as usual but is advised to keep their bowel moving to avoid barium impaction.

Risks

- Leakage of barium through an unsuspected perforation.
  - Intraperitoneal barium causes hypovolaemic shock and has a 50% mortality rate. Of those that survive, 30% have adhesions.
- Barium impaction (causing large bowel obstruction) or barium appendicitis.
- Medication effects (see 'other information').

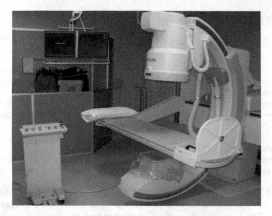

Fig. 6.4 A typical fluoroscopy room set up for an upper gastrointestinal barium examination.

Patient preparation

- Fasting: nil by mouth for 12 hours before the examination.
- Bowel preparation: laxative (usually Picolax® or similar) taken 12 hours before.

Other information

- Metoclopramide aids gastric emptying. Extra-pyramidal side effects may occur, especially in young women, and there is a risk of acute dystonic reactions such as an oculogyric crisis. Contraindicated in patients with Parkinsonism/Parkinson's disease.
- ▶ A barium study will prevent a CT examination of the same area for a period of time as intestinal barium creates dense streak artefact.

Barium enema

▶ The following refers to the standard 'double contrast' barium enema.

Indications

- Investigation of colonic pathology. Indications include pain, melaena, anaemia, palpable mass, change in bowel habit, failed colonoscopy, and investigation of remaining colon in the case of a known colonic tumour.
- ▶ Always consider alternatives (e.g. colonoscopy, CT colonography).

Contraindications

- Absolute: lack of informed consent, possible perforation, pseudomembranous colitis, toxic megacolon, biopsy via rigid sigmoidoscope within 5 days, biopsy via flexible endoscope within 1 day.
- Relative: barium meal within 7–14 days, patient frailty or immobility.
  - ▶ The procedure requires a large amount of patient cooperation. The patient must be able to lie flat and to turn over easily
  - ▶ The patient must be able to retain rectal barium and air.

Procedure

The colon is coated with barium, then inflated with air and images are taken from several different angles. Performed by a radiographer or radiologist.

- The patient lies in the left lateral position on the fluoroscopy table (Fig. 6.5).
- The operator may perform a digital rectal examination before starting.
- A rectal tube is placed, attached to a bag of barium sulphate. The barium is run into the colon under x-ray guidance until it reaches the right colon.
- The barium is drained.
- Intravenous buscopan or, if contraindicated, glucagon is given.
- The colon is inflated with air (or with CO_2 in some centres).
- The patient is instructed to roll and is tilted as images are acquired.
- Once the images are obtained, the colon is deflated and the patient can go to the bathroom to empty their bowel and shower if necessary.
- The examination may last 15–30 minutes.
- The patient should be kept in the department until any medication side effects (e.g. blurred vision) have worn off.

Risks

- Perforation (increased risk in elderly, ulcerating lesions, systemic steroids, hypothyroidism, large bowel obstruction).
  - Intraperitoneal barium causes hypovolaemic shock and has a 50% mortality rate. Of those that survive, 30% have adhesions.
- Cardiac arrhythmia (secondary to the large bowel distension).
- Medication effects (see 'other information').

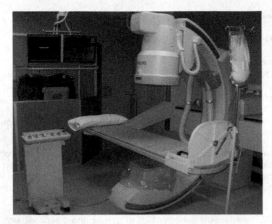

Fig. 6.5 A typical fluoroscopy room set up for a barium enema examination.

Patient preparation

- *Iron tablets:* stop 5 days before.
- *Constipating agents:* stop 2 days before.
- *Fasting:* low residue diet 2 days before, fluids only on the day before.
- *Bowel preparation:* laxative (usually Picolax®) taken at 08:00 and 18:00 on the day before.

Other information

- Buscopan is given to inhibit intestinal motility. Side effects include blurred vision, dry mouth, and tachycardia.
  - Contraindicated in angina, untreated closed angle glaucoma, prostatic hypertrophy, myasthenia gravis, paralytic ileus, pyloric stenosis
  - Glucagon is given if buscopan cannot be given. Risk of hypersensitivity and is contraindicated in phaeochromocytoma, insulinoma and glucagonoma.
- After the procedure, the patient may eat and drink as usual but is advised to keep their bowel moving to avoid barium impaction.
- ▶ A barium study will prevent a CT examination of the same area for a period of time as intestinal barium creates dense streak artefact.

Water-soluble contrast examinations

- In the case of recent surgery, suspected perforation, or investigation of a leak, water-based iodinated contrast is used instead of barium. Examples include Gastrograffin, Urograffin, Niopam, and Omnipaque.
- A single-contrast examination is performed (i.e. the colon is not inflated with air) and many of the 'standard' views are not included.
- No bowel preparation or fasting is needed.

Endoscopic retrograde cholangiopancreatography (ERCP)

Indications
- *Diagnostic:* largely superseded by safer modalities such as endoscopic ultrasound and MRI/MRCP. Diagnostic indications include sphincter of Oddi dysfunction and primary sclerosing cholangitis.
- *Therapeutic:* endoscopic sphincterotomy (biliary and pancreatic), removal of stones, dilation of strictures (e.g. PSC), stent placement.

Contraindications
- Lack of informed consent, uncooperative patient, recent attack of pancreatitis, recent MI, history of contrast dye anaphylaxis, severe cardiopulmonary disease, futility (anticipated short-term survival with no features of sepsis).

Procedure
An ERCP involves the passage of an endoscope into the duodenum. The endoscopist injects contrast medium through the ampulla of Vater via a catheter. Real-time fluoroscopy is used to visualize the pancreas and biliary tree. Selected images are taken.
- Dentures (if present) are removed.
- Patient is given anaesthetic throat spray (lidocaine) and sometimes intravenous sedation/analgesia (e.g. midazolam, pethidine).
- Patient lies on the couch in a modified left lateral ('swimmers') position with the left arm adducted and the right abducted. The endoscope is inserted as for OGD.
- Under x-ray guidance, a polyethylene catheter is inserted into the biliary tree and contrast instilled to outline the pancreatic duct as well as the common bile duct and its tributaries.
- Procedure time varies from 30–90 minutes.

Risks
- Pancreatitis (2–9% of procedures of which 10% of cases are mild–moderate). Serum amylase is temporarily raised in 70%.
- Infection (ascending cholangitis, acute cholecystitis, infected pancreatic pseudocyst, liver abscess, endocarditis).
- Bleeding, perforation of the oesophagus, duodenum, bile ducts.
- Failure of gallstone retrieval.
- Prolonged pancreatic stenting associated with stent occlusion, pancreatic duct obstruction, pseudocyst formation.
- Basket impaction around a large gallstone (may require surgery).

Patient preparation

- *Blood tests:* Liver enzymes, platelets, and clotting are checked prior to the procedure.
- *Fasting:* 4 hours except in the case of an emergency.
- *Antibiotic prophylaxis:* recommended for:
  - Patients in whom biliary decompression is unlikely to be achieved at a single procedure (e.g. dilatation of dominant stricture in multifocal sclerosing cholangitis or hilar cholangiocarcinoma)
  - Consider also in patients with severe neutropenia ($<0.5 \times 10^9$/L) and/or profound immunocompromise.

Other information

- ❶ Intravenous sedation and analgesia is usually administered and the back of the throat is sprayed with local anaesthetic.
- Hilar biliary obstruction demonstrated on MR or CT imaging may be more successfully stented using percutaneous transhepatic cholangiography (PTC) than ERCP.
- Equipment allowing direct cholangioscopy (with the potential for sampling lesions) is becoming more widely available.

Ultrasound

Indications
- Indications are manifold and too numerous to list. See 'making best use of a department of clinical radiology' via ♒ http://www.rcr.ac.uk

Contraindications
- For some examinations, the patient must be able to cooperate with the operator and a degree of mobility is often required.
- Ultrasound becomes increasingly less diagnostic at greater depths. Images of deeper structures in large individuals are often unobtainable and this should be borne in mind when considering who to refer.

Technology
- The ultrasound probe houses a piezoelectric crystal which both projects and receives high-frequency sound waves. Much like radar, the 'echoes' are converted to images by the machine's software.
- Ultrasound cannot image through gas and requires a semi-liquid 'gel' between the probe and skin surface for optimum imaging.
- A typical ultrasound machine is shown in Fig. 6.6.

Procedure
- This depends on the part of the body examined and the indications.
- Time taken will vary depending on part of body examined, patient cooperation, and complexity of the findings. Most examinations last between 5–20 minutes.

Risks
- ▶ There is no published evidence that ultrasound has ever directly caused harm to a patient.
  - The acoustic output of modern machines, however, is much greater than previously used.
- *Heating*: some equipment can produce temperature rises of 4°C in bone. Most equipment in clinical use is unlikely to increase tissue temperature more than the 1.5°C which is considered 'safe'.
- *Non-thermal hazard:* ultrasound has been demonstrated to produce tiny gas pockets and bubbles in animal models. Neonatal lung is considered vulnerable to this but there is no evidence that diagnostic ultrasound can cause harm to other tissues.
  - Machines have a 'mechanical index' (MI) displayed on screen which acts as a guide to the operator.

Patient preparation
Depends on the indication and body part being examined.
- *Abdomen:* patients are usually asked to fast for 6 hours prior to the examination. This ensures distension of the gallbladder and prevents the epigastric structures being obscured by overlying bowel gas.
- *Renal tract/pelvis:* a full bladder is usually required. A full bladder creates an 'acoustic window', effectively pushing small bowel aside so that deeper structures (e.g. ovaries) may be seen.

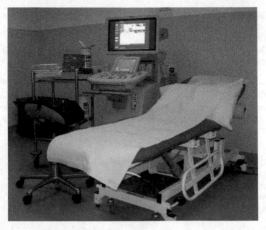

Fig. 6.6 A typical ultrasound room.

Oesophagogastroduodenoscopy (OGD)

Indications

- *Diagnostic:* haematemesis, dyspepsia (>55 years old), oesophageal and gastric biopsies (malignancy?), duodenal biopsies (coeliac?), surveillance (e.g. Barrett's oesophagus), persistent nausea and vomiting, iron-deficiency anaemia, dysphagia.
- *Therapeutic:* treatment of bleeding lesions, variceal banding and sclerotherapy, stricture dilatation, polypectomy, EMR, palliative intent (e.g. stent insertion, laser therapy), argon plasma coagulation for suspected vascular lesions.

Contraindications

- *Absolute:* lack of informed consent, possible perforation, haemodynamic instability, hypoxaemia with respiratory distress, uncooperative patient.
- *Relative:* pharyngeal diverticulum, recent myocardial infarction, or pulmonary embolus.

Procedure

- Endoscopic examination of the mucosa of the oesophagus, stomach, and proximal duodenum. Allows direct visualization, mucosal biopsies, and other therapeutic procedures.
- Dentures (if present) are removed.
- Patient is given anaesthetic throat spray (lidocaine) +/− intravenous sedation (e.g. midazolam).
- Patient lies on the couch in the left lateral position.
- Hollow mouthpiece is inserted to protect the patient's teeth and facilitate instrument passage.
- Endoscope (9.5–12.5mm diameter, max 120cm long) is slowly advanced and 'swallowed' by the patient (Fig. 6.7 shows a typical scope).
- Scope advanced and manipulated by the endoscopist to allow visualization of the target structures.
- Procedure time varies but averages 5–15 minutes.

Risks

- Minor throat and abdominal discomfort.
- Cardiorespiratory: arrthythmias, MI, respiratory arrest, shock, death.
- Infection (uncommon, e.g. aspiration pneumonia).
- Perforation (around 0.03% with a mortality of 0.001% during diagnostic procedures, higher with therapeutic procedures).
  - Overall 2–3% perforation with oesophageal dilatation; mortality 1%.
- Bleeding (caution with low platelet counts and high INR).
- Medication effects including anaphylactic reactions and over-sedation.
- Dental trauma.

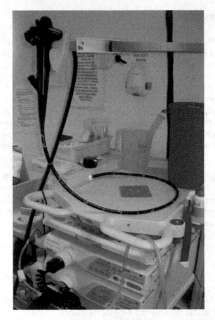

Fig. 6.7 A typical gastroscope.

Patient preparation

- *Fasting:* 4 hours prior to the procedure unless in an emergency situation.
- *Antibiotic prophylaxis:* none for OGD. See other topics for comparison.

Other information

- Dosages of benzodiazepines and opiates should be kept to a minimum to achieve sedation, with lower doses being prescribed in elderly patients.
- The pharynx is sprayed with local anaesthetic spray. There is some evidence that the combination use of local anaesthetic spray and intravenous sedation increases the risk of aspiration pneumonia.
- ❶ Patients who have had intravenous sedation should not drive, operate heavy machinery, or drink alcohol for 24 hours afterwards.

Colonoscopy

Indications

- *Diagnostic:* gastrointestinal bleeding, iron-deficiency anaemia, chronic diarrhoea, lower abdominal symptoms (chronic constipation, lower abdominal pain, bloating), evaluation of known IBD, surveillance for cancer (in IBD patients/after colonic polypectomy/after curative intent resection of colorectal cancer), screening for colorectal cancer.
- *Therapeutic:* polypectomy (including endoscopic mucosal resection techniques: EMR), angiodysplasia treated with argon plasma coagulation (APC), decompression of volvulus or pseudo-obstruction, dilatation or stenting of strictures or malignant colonic obstruction.

Contraindications

- *Absolute:* lack of informed consent, toxic megacolon, fulminant colitis, colonic perforation.
- *Relative:* acute diverticulitis, symptomatic large abdominal aortic aneurysm, immediately post-op, recent myocardial infarction or pulmonary embolus, severe coagulopathies.
  - Colonoscopy can be performed safely in pregnancy but should be deferred in most instances unless requiring immediate resolution.

Procedure

Colonoscopy is an endoscopic examination of the mucosal surface from the anal canal to the terminal ileum.

- Patient lies on the couch in the left lateral position with knees bent.
- Endoscopist first performs a digital rectal examination.
- Sedation (e.g. midazolam) may be given with monitoring of oxygen saturation. Intravenous analgesia (e.g. pethidine) is also given.
  - Increasing use of either no sedation (with improved techniques such as 'Scopeguide®') or inhaled nitric oxide.
- Lubricated colonoscope (about 12mm wide and 185cm long) is passed rectally. Air is insufflated. Water-jet may also be used via the scope.
  - Figure 6.8 shows a typical scope.
- Aim is to pass to the terminal ileum.
- Duration varies but averages at about 20 minutes.

Risks

- Perforation (0.2–0.4% diagnostic; higher with therapeutic procedures).
- Bleeding (1 in 1000).
- Abdominal distension, medication effects (allergic reactions, nausea, vomiting hypotension, respiratory depression).
- Rarities: infection, post-polypectomy coagulation syndrome: pain, peritoneal irritation, leukocytosis and fever, splenic rupture, small bowel obstruction.

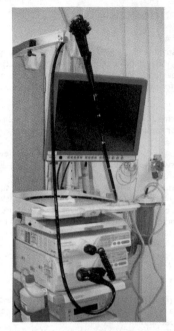

Fig. 6.8 A typical colonoscope.

Patient preparation

- *Iron and constipating agents:* discontinue iron tablets 7 days and constipating agents 4 days prior to the procedure.
- *Anticoagulant and antiplatelet therapy:* in the case of a planned polypectomy or other therapeutic procedure, refer to BSG guidelines on the management of anticoagulant and antiplatelet therapy: ✍ http://www.bsg.org.uk.
- *Antibiotic prophylaxis:* none for colonoscopy. See other topics for comparison.
- *Bowel preparation:* the colon must be empty. Protocols vary but usually include prescribing 1 sachet of sodium picosulphate (Picolax®) for the morning and afternoon of the day before procedure.

Other information

- The introduction of the bowel cancer screening programme has meant that endoscopists need to pass a 'driving test' to demonstrate high-level competency to perform safe screening colonoscopy.
- Endoscopic mucosal resection (EMR) is used for larger or difficult flat polyps. The lesion is lifted by submucosal injection of gelofusin, adrenaline, and dye followed by snare resection. Polyps can then be retrieved by 'Roth' baskets for histological assessment.

Capsule endoscopy

Indications

- Obscure gastrointestinal bleeding (in patients with negative gastroscopy and ileocolonoscopy), known or suspected small bowel Crohn's disease, assessment of coeliac disease, screening and surveillance for polyps in familial polyposis syndromes.

Contraindications

- Lack of informed consent, intestinal strictures, adhesions, obstruction.
- Diverticula or fistulae that may block the passage of capsule endoscope.
- Cardiac pacemakers or other implanted electronic devices.
- Difficulty in swallowing tablets or known swallowing disorders.
- Pregnancy (lack of available safety data).
- ▶ Patients with obstructive symptoms or known or suspected inflammatory bowel disease should have either a small bowel follow through or a patency capsule (dissolves after 36 hours), with an abdominal radiograph taken 24 hours post ingestion to identify whether capsule is retained within small bowel.
  - If retained, capsule endoscopy is not appropriate
  - ▶ Capsule retention can occur even in the absence of strictures on barium or MR-enteroclysis study.

Procedure

- The capsule (Fig. 6.9) consists of a disposable, wireless, miniature video camera which can be swallowed and passes through the intestine by peristalsis.
- Images taken by the capsule are transmitted, via sensors secured to the abdominal wall, to a battery-powered data recorder worn on a belt.
- The capsule leaves the stomach within 30 mins and the patient is allowed to drink after 2 hours and eat after 4 hours.
- The external equipment (Fig. 6.10) is removed after 8 hours (approximate battery life) by which time the capsule has reached the caecum in 85% of patients.
- The capsule is expelled naturally after 24–48 hours in the patient's stool and does not need to be collected.
- Data from the recorder is downloaded onto a computer workstation which allows approximately 50,000 images to be viewed as a video.

Risks

- Capsule retention (may cause partial or complete intestinal obstruction; highest risk in patients with extensive small bowel Crohn's disease, chronic usage of NSAIDs, abdominal radiation injury, previous major abdominal surgery, or small bowel resection).
- Capsule endoscopy may also fail in patients with dysphagia, gastroparesis, and anatomical abnormalities of the gastrointestinal tract.

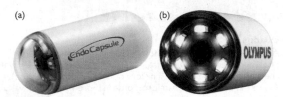

Fig. 6.9 Examples of a typical capsule endoscope. It is shaped to be easy to swallow and has its own light-source.

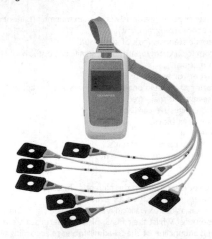

Fig. 6.10 The external equipment which the patient will wear, consisting of a data-recorder and electrodes.

Patient preparation
- *Iron supplements:* stop taking 1 week prior to procedure.
- *Constipating agents:* stop 4 days before the procedure.
- *Fasting:* patients are fasted for 8–12 hours prior to the procedure and may receive bowel prep (taken day before procedure).

Other information
- Incomplete examination in 10–25% of cases.
  - Presence of dark intestinal contents in distal small bowel may impair visualization of mucosa
  - Delayed gastric emptying and small bowel transit can lead to exhaustion of battery life before capsule reaches ileocaecal valve.
- Capsules are being developed to screen for oesophageal varices and may be more 'guided' in future as the technology develops.
- Positive findings on capsule endoscopy may be reachable using either single- or double-balloon enteroscopy or spiral enteroscopy.

Exercise tolerance test (ETT)

Indications
- Assessment of chest pain in those with known coronary artery disease (there is no longer a role for ETT in patients presenting with chest pain who do not have a history of coronary artery disease).
- Assessment of haemodynamic response in those with known valvular disease who are asymptomatic.
- Diagnosis of exertionally induced arrhythmias or syncope.

Contraindications
- Any undiagnosed or previously unknown murmur (patient should undergo echocardiogram first).
- Severe aortic stenosis (risk of syncope).
- Hypertrophic cardiomyopathy with significant outflow obstruction (risk of syncope).
- Severe hyper- or hypo-tension.
- Unstable angina (should undergo coronary angiography).
- Known severe left main stem disease.
- Untreated congestive cardiac failure.
- Complete heart block.
- Aortic aneurysm.
- Acute myocarditis or pericarditis.
- Any recent pyrexial or 'flu-like' illness.

Procedure
- ECG electrodes are put on the patient's chest and a sphygmomanometer cuff on an arm.
- The patient is asked to walk on a treadmill (see Fig. 6.11) connected to the computer whilst their ECG, BP, and heart rate are monitored. The speed and incline of the treadmill increase according to set protocols:
  - Bruce protocol: for assessment of physically fit and stable patients with suspected coronary artery disease. Seven stages starting at a 10% gradient at 1.7mph and increasing to 22% gradient and 6mph
  - Modified Bruce protocol: used in elderly patients or those who have been stabilized after a suspected episode of unstable angina. Starts at 1.7mph and 0% gradient and increases the gradient slowly to 10%.
- Termination of the test depends on the results seen.

Risks
- Risks are those associated with exercise and include:
  - Arrhythmia, cardiac ischaemia, myocardial infarction, syncope.

Patient preparation
- No specific preparation is required.
- Patients are asked not to eat or drink for 3 hours prior to the test.
- Comfortable clothing and shoes should be worn.

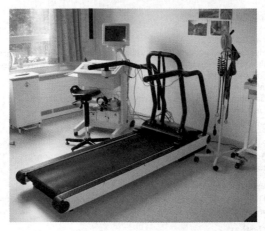

Fig. 6.11 A typical ETT room.

Indications for termination of procedure
- Patient requests to stop.
- *Symptoms:* fatigue, angina, dizziness, significant breathlessness.
- *Signs:* drop in oxygen saturations <94%, target heart rate achieved, hypotension during exercise (e.g. BP <100mmHg), significant hypertension (e.g. BP >200mmHg).
- *ECG:* any atrial or ventricular arrhythmia, frequent ventricular ectopics, new AV or bundle branch block, ST segment shift >1mm.

Causes of false positive results or low specificity
- Often due to difficulty interpreting results as result of resting ST segment abnormalities:
  - Wolff–Parkinson–White syndrome, LBBB, atrial fibrillation, left ventricular hypertrophy, digoxin therapy, hyperventilation, biochemical electrolyte abnormalities (e.g. hypo- or hyperkalaemia), cardiomyopathies, LV outflow obstruction.
- Beta-blocker therapy prevents the appropriate heart rate/blood pressure response during testing.

Echocardiography

Indications
- Myocardial infarction: assess wall motion and left ventricular function.
- Valvular heart disease: assess competency and examine prostheses.
- Embolic stroke: to exclude a cardiac embolic source.
- Infective endocarditis: look for valvular vegetations.
- Cardiomyopathy: assess ventricular dilatation/hypertrophy and function.
- Congenital heart disease.
- Pericardial disease.
- Pericardial effusion: distribution of fluid and suitability for drainage.
- Aortic disease: severity and site of aneurysm, dissection, or coarctation.

Contraindications
- The only contraindication is lack of patient consent or if the patient is unable to cooperate.

Technology
- Echocardiography is an ultrasound examination and uses the same technology (and machines) as general ultrasound (Fig. 6.12).
- Ultrasound becomes increasingly less diagnostic at greater depths and cannot see through lung. Images in large individuals are often suboptimal and the heart may not be seen at all in patients with hyperinflated lungs.
- See Box 6.1 for other types.

Procedure
- Time taken will vary depending on examinations performed and complexity of the findings.
- Most examinations last between 20–25 minutes.
- With the patient lying on their left side, the operator uses a hand-held probe coated with gel to examine the heart usually via the anterior chest and epigastrium.

Risks
- ▶ There is no published evidence that ultrasound has ever directly caused any harm to a patient.
- *Heating:* some equipment can produce temperature rises of 4°C in bone. Most equipment in clinical use is unlikely to increase tissue temperature more than the 1.5°C which is considered 'safe'.
- *Non-thermal hazard:* ultrasound has been demonstrated to produce tiny gas pockets and bubbles in animal models but there is no evidence that diagnostic ultrasound can cause harm to tissues other than neonatal lung.

Patient preparation
- No preparation is required.

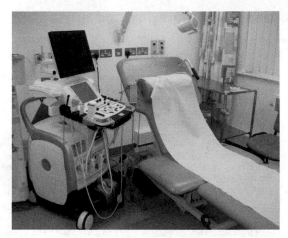

Fig. 6.12 A typical echocardiography room.

Box 6.1 Other types of echocardiography

Along with 2-dimensional trans-thoracic echocardiography, the following methods exist:

- *3D:* uses computer software to produce a 3-dimensional image. Useful in left-ventricular functional assessment especially post-infarction
- *4D:* 3D imaging with real-time movement captured
- *TOE:* trans-oesophageal echo is an invasive procedure. It requires written consent and is performed under sedation with local anaesthetic spray to the upper pharynx. The probe is covered, lubricated, and passed into the oesophagus behind the heart. It is used to visualize the posterior cardiac structures. The investigation of choice for infective endocarditis
- *Stress echo:* Used to assess myocardial ischaemia at 'rest' and during 'stress'. Stress is induced by exercise or (more commonly) by an intravenous infusion of dobutamine in a controlled environment
- *Bubble studies:* Used to assess for intra-cardiac shunts such as atrial or ventricular septal defects or patent foramen ovale. Air bubbles are agitated in a syringe and injected into a peripheral vein. The Valsalva manoeuvre is performed and, if a shunt exists, bubbles will be seen moving from the right side of the heart to the left.

Coronary angiography and angioplasty

Indications

- *Diagnostic:* unstable or refractory angina, acute coronary syndrome, positive or inconclusive stress testing.
- *Emergency therapeutic:* where possible, patients presenting with acute ST-elevation myocardial infarction should have primary coronary intervention rather than thrombolysis.
- *Elective therapeutic:* suitable 'target lesion' identified on diagnostic coronary angiogram.

Contraindications

- *Absolute:* refusal of patient consent.
- *Relative:* acute renal failure, pulmonary oedema, known radiographic contrast allergy, uncontrolled hypertension, active GI haemorrhage, acute stroke, and untreated coagulopathy.

Procedure

- A typical cardiac interventional suite is shown in Fig. 6.13.
- Percutaneous access via a guide needle into a peripheral artery (most commonly the radial artery).
- Guide catheter is introduced, the tip is placed at the coronary ostium, radio-opaque contrast is injected, and real-time x-ray is used to visualize the blood flow through the coronary arteries.
- The coronary guidewire is inserted through the catheter into the coronary artery using x-ray guidance.
- The guidewire tip is passed across the site of stenosis.
- The balloon catheter is passed over the guidewire until the deflated balloon lies across the target lesion.
- The balloon is then inflated and compresses the plaque and stretches the artery wall. A stent (wire mesh tube) can be inserted using a similar technique and be left in place maintaining the arterial lumen.
- The guidewire, catheter, and sheath are carefully removed.
- The patient should remain supine for 4 hours following the procedure unless an arterial closure device has been used.

Risks

- *Minor:* contrast allergy, vasovagal reaction, haemorrhage and haematoma at puncture site, thrombosis formation, false aneurysm, arteriovenous fistulation, pulmonary oedema, and renal failure due to contrast nephropathy.
- *Major:* limb ischaemia, coronary artery dissection, aortic dissection, ventricular perforation, air or atheroma embolism, ventricular arrhythmias, failure of procedure and need to proceed to CABG.
- Death (<1 in 1000).

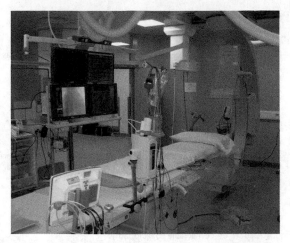

Fig. 6.13 A typical cardiac interventional suite.

Patient preparation

- Pre-procedure checklist: written consent, group and save, ECG, check FBC/clotting/urea and electrolytes.

Other information

- Coronary angioplasty is associated with increased thrombus formation (balloon inflation disrupts the intima, revealing pro-thrombotic cores of plaques), therefore antiplatelet therapy is necessary.
- Patients will need to have long-term antiplatelet therapy; usually lifelong aspirin 75mg od, but they will also need clopidogrel 75mg od (see local guidelines: usually 3 months for bare metal stents and 12 months for drug-eluting stents or angioplasty after acute coronary syndrome).
- Patients with renal failure should be carefully considered. Iodinated contrast can be nephrotoxic and renal decompensation may occur following coronary angiography/plasty. The risk can be minimized by hydration before and after the procedure. Renal function should be carefully monitored. Check local guidelines.

Bronchoscopy

Indications

- *Diagnostic:* histology/cytology in suspected lung malignancy, sample mediastinal lymphadenopathy, alveolar lavage (e.g. tuberculosis), transbronchial biopsy (e.g. diffuse lung disease).
- *Therapeutic:* placement of guidewire for local radiotherapy, direct treatment (e.g. diathermy to strictures).
  - Placement of endobronchial stents and the removal of foreign bodies are usually accomplished at rigid bronchoscopy under GA.

Contraindications

- *Absolute:* cardiovascular instability, life-threatening arrhythmia, severe hypoxaemia, respiratory failure with hypercapnia (unless intubated/ ventilated).
  - *Rigid bronchoscopy contraindications:* unstable neck, severely ankylosed cervical spine, severely restricted temporomandibular joints.
- *Relative:* uncooperative patient, recent myocardial infarction, tracheal obstruction, un-correctable coagulopathy.
  - Transbronchial biopsy with caution in uraemia, SVCO, pulmonary hypertension (risk of bleeding).

Procedure

Bronchoscopy is an endoscopic examination of the bronchial tree.

- Patient sits on the couch, leaning back comfortably.
- Sedation (e.g. midazolam) may be given with monitoring of oxygen saturation. Atropine may also be given to decrease secretions.
- Pharynx is anaesthetized with aerosolized lidocaine.
- Lubricated bronchoscope (about 6mm wide and 60cm long) is passed nasally or orally with use of a bite-block (Fig. 6.14).
- Brushings, biopsy, or lavage (50–100ml saline) may be performed.
- Duration varies but averages about 20–30 minutes.

Risks

- Bleeding from a biopsy site and transient fever (10–15%).
- Medication effects: respiratory depression, hypotension, arrhythmias.
- Topical anaesthesia: laryngospasm, bronchospasm, seizures, arrhythmias.
- Minor laryngeal oedema or injury with hoarseness, hypoxaemia in patients with compromised gas exchange (1–10%).
- Mortality is 1–4 in 10,000 patients.
- Transbronchial biopsy: pneumothorax (2–5%), significant haemorrhage (1%); death (12 in 10,000).

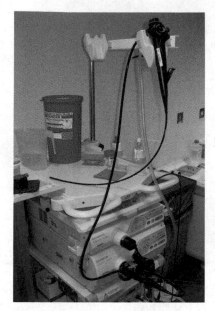

Fig. 6.14 A typical bronchoscope.

Patient preparation

- *Anticoagulant and antiplatelet therapy:* stop for 3 days. Clopidogrel should be stopped for 5 days.
- *Blood tests:* check clotting and full blood count.
- *Spirometry:* perform if underlying lung disease.
- *Fasting:* nil by mouth 2 hours before the procedure, no solids 4–6 hours before procedure.

Post-procedure

- *Oxygen:* supplemental oxygen for up to 1 hour.
- *Eating/drinking:* drink after 1 hour. If no problems, can eat.
- *Chest radiography:* only if dyspnoea or chest pain following biopsy (10% risk of pneumothorax).
- *Driving:* if had midazolam or similar, not to drive or operate heavy machinery for the rest of the day.

Index